I've known Peter for twenty years, first as a strength coach for the Seattle Reign—Seattle's first women's professional basketball team—and more recently as my personal trainer. Peter possesses a special combination of experience, skills, and demeanor that allows him to reach and positively impact people of all walks of life—from an elite athlete to a middle-aged woman trying to get fit again. His approach is methodical, disciplined, and holistic, while also being practical, realistic, and fun. Peter is an inspirational teacher, and my time with him has been a true gift.

—KAREN BRYANT, FORMER GENERAL MANAGER, SEATTLE REIGN AND PRESIDENT & CEO, SEATTLE STORM

A Life Athlete is who we all become at some point. Acknowledge it, embrace it, live it, and learn from it to become the best and healthiest life athlete you know! Set high goals and chase them. Peter's book will set you on the course to doing so.

— JAMIE MOYER, FORMER MAJOR LEAGUE BASEBALL PLAYER AND OLDEST PITCHER TO WIN A MLB GAME, AT 49.

Shmock's search for excellence in throwing a 16 lb. iron ball farther than anyone in the world led to a search for completeness as a person. The lessons he shares about learning and growing are not just for Olympic competition, but for life.

— MAC WILKINS, FOUR-TIME US OLYMPIC TEAM MEMBER (DISCUS THROW), OLYMPIC GOLD MEDALIST IN 1976

These valuable lessons have made me think differently about training and movement. Shmock's strategies for keeping physically healthy and active have resonance in my daily life as a business person and father. They serve as a template for how to approach any big challenge in life.

— PETER BAILEY, CEO OF VERTICAL COMMUNICATIONS, PRINCETON FOOTBALL PLAYER, MASTERS CYCLIST, FATHER, HUSBAND, ETC.

A lifetime of tools and language to help us feel more alive, no matter what age.

A compelling and edifying story of the challenges, struggles, victories, and triumphs faced by a world class athlete. Peter Shmock writes *The Life Athlete* in a friendly, congenial voice, as if he's telling us a few ideas over a sandwich and a cup of coffee at the neighborhood deli, and in this approachable manner, Peter reveals many important lessons he has learned: while athletics are important, athletics aren't all; the well-being of our bodies is dependent on the well-being of our minds and our spirits, and vice versa; living the life of the athlete does not include a finish line—the race in which we participate is a lifetime long. Peter elevates the discussion of 'getting in shape' from being about a person's body, to encompassing a person's mind and soul. *The Life Athlete* is a must read for all who are alive and have a body.

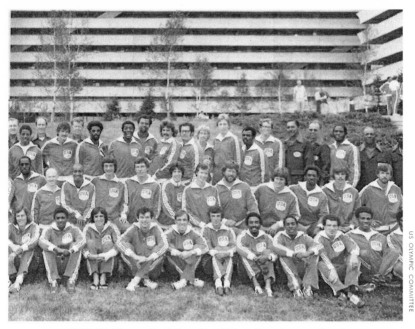

1976 US Olympic Track Team (I'm fifth from the right, second row)

THE WAY OF
THE LIFE ATHLETE

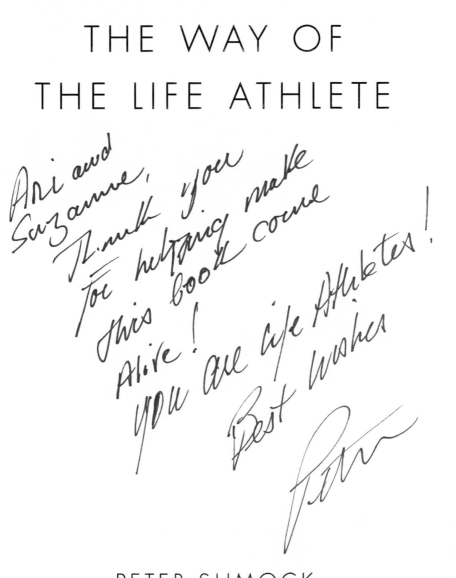

Ari and Suzanne,
Thank you for helping make this book come Alive!
You are Life Athletes!
Best wishes
Peter

PETER SHMOCK

Shmock, Peter
The Way of the Life Athlete
ISBN 978-0-9976565-0-3

1. Biography & Autobiography—Sports. 2. Health & Fitness—Healthy Living.
3. Body, Mind & Spirit—Inspiration & Personal Growth. 4. Self-Help—Personal
Growth & Success. 5. Sports & Recreation—Training.

Drawings by Peter Shmock
Book design by Sayre Coombs
Cover photo: Eugene Register-Guard
Author photo: Oliver Ludlow

Permission to reprint photo of the 1976 US Olympic Track and Field Team is
granted by the US Olympic Committee.

Printed in the United States of America

THE WAY OF
THE LIFE ATHLETE

TABLE OF CONTENTS

Living the life of the athlete does not
include a finish line—the race in which we
participate is a lifetime long

GARTH STEIN

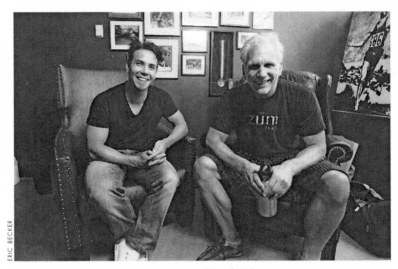

Hanging out with Apolo Ohno

FOREWORD
by Apolo Ohno

Not so long ago, I competed in short track speed skating. I had set my sights on some really big goals, and I pushed myself to the max in order to achieve them. Back then, when gold medals were on the line, I'd train crazy hard from dawn till dusk, eat a pizza, and bounce back just fine the next day. Such is the glory of youth.

At home in Seattle on my occasional breaks from training, I wanted to do something different from my normal, strenuous routine, something quieter and more mellow. So I followed my dad's recommendation and called Peter Shmock. When I met him in the early 2000s, we instantly connected. Both of us had our interest in athletics sparked at an early age and spent our formative years pursuing it. Both of us had the honor of going to the Olympic Games (for different sports and a few decades apart, of course). But it was his philosophy that got me, his focus on more mindful, meditative styles of training, his continual insistence that training doesn't have to be an exercise in ballistic *ass-kicker-y* to be effective.

As I got older and more experienced in my sport, I began to notice that a lot of elite athletes—myself included—tended to overdo it, to use a blowtorch when a lighter would work just as well. And I began to see a pattern of training styles among those who burned out versus those who made progress. *Surprise, surprise:* Usually the guys on the podium were the ones who took a more moderate approach.

There was something else about Peter that I could only appreciate after my own retirement from world competition-level athletics. Peter had made that difficult transition from professional athlete to regular-yet-super-fit guy, from someone who lives to train to someone who trains to live. He'd spent years and years living, breathing, sleeping, and eating sports training, fitness, and other health-focused forms of life training. Now, he has a lot to show for it. He can help the top 1 percent of the top 1 percent of elite athletes, those who are in their competitive prime, reach peak performance. That's a particular breed with particular needs, and yet Peter has figured out a way to adapt that system to work just as well for folks who want to be fit and healthy in a normal kind of way, who want to feel good in their bodies and look good, too.

We all have important things to do, whether it's paying our bills, lowering our cholesterol, raising our kids, or working out (because nice pecs don't grow on trees). Peter's *The Way of the Life Athlete* is meant to support all the obligations and activities you have and do, to get you healthy and/or keep you healthy for as long as humanly possible. In this book, you'll find not only the story of his Olympic achievements and beyond, but also some great insights and no-nonsense advice gleaned from the many awesome teachers and challenging experiences he encountered along the way.

Whether you're reading The Way of the Life Athlete *on the treadmill, in your post-workout ice bath, or while waiting for your double-pepperoni pizza to arrive, you'll find something that'll work for you, your body, and your life.*

PROLOGUE

've been training people for more than thirty-five years. Before that, I was an Olympic athlete, competing in the shot put event in the 1976 Olympics and 1980 Olympic Trials. I've spent my life trying to figure out how the imperfect machine of the body/mind works best, and using whatever lucky insights I've gleaned along the way to help others.

In more recent years, I had the good fortune to work with Ken Russell, a gifted and caring teacher of meditation and other practices of self-awareness. He gave me the great gift of advocacy, and with his encouragement I began to learn how to pay attention. He nudged me hard toward a better awareness of my decisions—my assumptions, my blind stumbling, my contribution to my own suffering—and he showed me that life could be good if I was willing to work for it.

Ken was not a person easy to fool, and he wasn't afraid to call bullshit as he saw it or tell people a truth they didn't want to hear. He once shared with me a conversation he'd had with a prospective student. After a few minutes talking on the phone with this guy, Ken told him, "I can't help you. You are satisfied with your life as it is. It's clear to me that you don't want anything better."

I'm guessing that, because you've picked up this book, you're either curious about how to become an Olympic shot-putter, or you're looking for something. If it's the former, then I hope that my story will ignite a desire within you to seek beyond where you are today. If it's the latter, then I hope I can help you in your quest. So: welcome. You're in the right place.

Desire is the first and most important step for the life athlete. Of course, that's not enough. Sorry. It takes a lot of work being alive, and it takes even more work being alive and doing it well. So how can you live well? There are a lot of opinions out there, and a lot of people who are more than willing to tell you them. Here comes the second part of the process: figure out where unexamined dogma exists in your life, and then examine it.

If you take a look around, you might notice that the norm doesn't work for everyone. It certainly works for some, or else why would it be so popular? All I know is, it certainly didn't work for me, and if you're here, something about it probably isn't working for you. Old, unexamined habits are deadweight—all they do is slow you down. As you begin to look for something different—something better—you have to decide what's no longer helpful and then let it go. Alas, this is not an easy process and there is no quick fix; observing your ingrained conditioning and figuring out how to shed that weight is a long-haul deal.

If you've seen *The Matrix,* this is that moment where Neo has to choose between the red pill and the blue pill. The blue pill will let him live in safe ignorance; the red pill will open his eyes to the truth. And the truth ain't pretty. Every day, we have this same—albeit less dramatic—choice. That moves us into the next phase: giving yourself permission to fully commit to the seeking. At this point, you can't be complacent anymore. You're not satisfied with something, and now you have to face that immense sea of all that you don't know and jump right in.

Trust is the thing that will build you a life raft, both in trusting yourself—your intelligence and your intuition—and in your ability to find something outside yourself that is worth trusting. A smart teacher, a well-researched article, a wise mentor, a timely fortune cookie, a kind friend. A book.

I very much hope that I've been able to capture my sixty-odd years of experience and intentional practice on these pages, and that you might find that what I've come up with resonates or, better yet, helps.

Welcome to The Way of the Life Athlete.

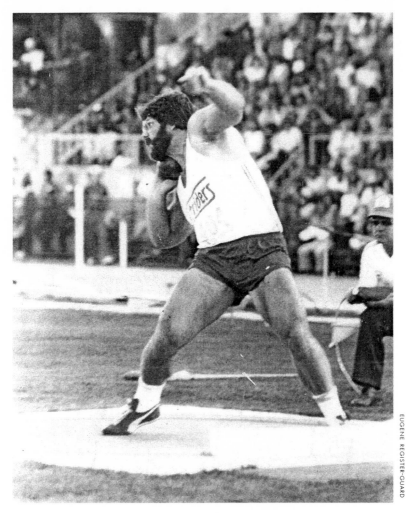

US Olympic Trials, 1980

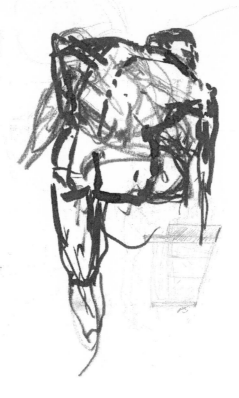

If you're going to try, go all the way.
Otherwise don't even start.
There's no feeling like that.
You will be alone with the gods,
and the nights will flame with fire.
You will ride life straight to perfect laughter.
It's the only fight there is.

CHARLES BUKOWSKI

FINDING GRIT

Superman was bad ass. Faster than a speeding bullet. More powerful than a locomotive. Able to leap tall buildings in a single bound. Superhuman Superman was a true superhero.

When I was a kid, I watched *The Adventures of Superman,* mesmerized. He was, and always will be, the shit. But I wasn't just fascinated with his daring feats of strength and speed. What I admired most about him was his clarity of mind and that when he used it, he could do anything. In a way, you might say those moments in front of the television started me on the path of my athletic career and, ultimately, the path of the Life Athlete. Though I don't possess Superman's Kryptonian body or skill set, I have spent a lifetime trying to follow in his footsteps by developing my mind in order to fully live out my potential. In a nutshell, Superman showed me what it means to have grit.

"Grit" is a hot word these days: "Our kids will be fine if they have grit!" "Our athletes will get the gold if they have grit!" But what, exactly, is behind this buzzword? I think of grit as all-encompassing: It is the strength and will to overcome the struggles we face, not only in our bodies but in the effort to make a better life. Grit is coming back again and again, refocusing and recommitting despite setbacks or heartache. Grit is what it takes to go beyond self-doubt, situational hardship, and bodily limitations.

As you move toward a goal, you will meet resistance, and here's where grit comes in. At some point we all succumb to self-doubt, confusion, and catastrophic thinking. We may feel hopeless, that whatever we had envisioned will be forever out of reach. But anything worth doing brings with it an assortment of doubts and concerns—these may even be signs that we are on the right track. This is just a natural part of the process. Having grit allows us to face negative thinking and to weaken its hold on our confidence.

For example, let's say you want to create a much-needed lifestyle shift around your health. You'd like to change your diet and exercise regimen. At first, it's difficult; you've developed some inertia around this kind of discipline. So in order to make these changes, you must find the grit necessary to practice your new lifestyle. Regardless of your starting point, it's essential to keep at it day after day. Of course you'll go off-course—a few donuts here or there, a skipped workout, a late night, the body's inevitable aches or injuries, a despairing thought. These set-backs are perfect for testing your grit—to allow you the opportunity to pick up where you left off once those moments pass. If you can press on through hardship and doubt, your efforts will gain momentum.

This chapter is about finding the grit within, despite limiting beliefs and doubt, and using that grit to get us to places we didn't think we could reach. We need grit to make us better, to win the race, to change our lives, and to attain higher levels of self-actualization. But how we get it, learn it, and cultivate it can come from many places. We can develop it through hardship (in many cases kicking and screaming at the world as we go). We can learn by example, from seeing the dis-cipline of parents, members of the community, great historical figures we admire, or coaches, mentors, and guides we stumble across when we least expect it. In my case, a comic book character—the badass Superman—ignited a fire in me that sparked a profound desire to train my mind and to excel athletically. Of course, Superman couldn't take me by the hand and lead the way—but my first human teacher of the "Superman way" could, and his name was Ralph Kroger.

INITIATION INTO GRIT WITH RALPH KROGER

I met Ralph at the end of my freshman year of high school. Ralph owned the Pacific Coast Health Studio, a small health club in Solana Beach, California. At that time—in the mid-1960s—weight training was mostly done by men for bodybuilding purposes. Gyms where body-builders congregated were few and far between, and they were seldom open to the average Joe or Jane who might want to pursue weight train-ing for purely health and fitness reasons.

Despite this, Ralph was able to attract a wide range of people to his gym—men and women, multi-sport athletes, and highly focused varsity teams. I didn't know it then, but this was the first time that luck would land me in a like-minded community, a community that was willing to spend time, money, and effort to improve themselves both physically and mentally.

Ralph was an up-and-coming bodybuilder then. He later went on to compete numerous times in the Mr. America competition, placing fourth in his best year. He was noted for his discipline, quiet strength, and his dedication to spreading his vision of health and fitness. He stood at 5'9" and weighed around 200 lb., though around contest time he would lean up to 185 lb. or so. He was a former paratrooper and though often serious, he could also laugh and joke with the gym members. He set the mood at the club: serious but not rigid, with a vibe of lightness that countered the cold-steel weights.

Occasionally we would see him eating multiple cans of tuna fish to get the protein he needed to increase muscular size and reduce body fat. He never talked about himself and would never work out in public view. His workouts were always behind locked doors, early in the morning before he opened the gym for the rest for us. He occasionally took on training partners, lesser body builders that he would invite to lift with him. These partners were a small and select few. I eventually became one of those invited to join him, and I'll never forget the experience of watching him at work.

I remember the first morning that I worked out with Ralph. It was still dark outside, and the gym was empty and quiet. Without any sort of warmup, he said, "Let's work biceps and triceps." Ralph went first, choosing the bicep movement, and he got up to ten or twelve repetitions until he couldn't do another one. He did the last few reps in each set with a stoicism that I will never be able to fully explain. He didn't grunt or groan or make facial expressions; he put every available ounce of energy into each rep until there was nothing left. *Unfuckingbelievable,* I thought. *Absolute focus and concentration* without a peep. I had never seen that before. His mind drove his body to the limit each and every time without regard to the strain he was feeling. This was my introduction to grit in action. His phrase *"put your mind to it"* sparked my *"gotta wanna"*—my deep desire and drive toward reaching a higher level of achievement.

Ralph created all of my weight-lifting programs for the three years I trained with him. I didn't just work out at Pacific Coast Health

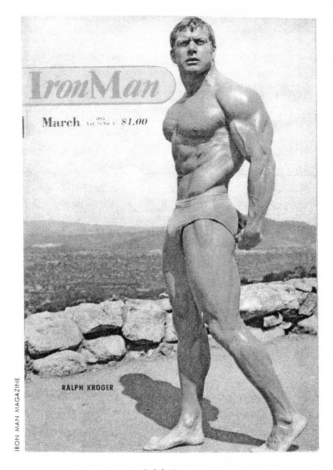

Ralph Kroger

Studio, I basically lived there. I'd train four to five days a week for up to three hours at a time. The workouts he created included vintage body-building moves that worked every single muscle and muscle group from calves to forearms, with the sublime athletic lifts that build whole body strength. I learned power cleans and squats, and I used these foundational movements over the course of my athletic career and beyond. Pacific Coast Health Studios was more like a school than a gym—a university of physical culture and mental education. And the headmaster was Professor Kroger.

In order to become stronger, I had to lift more weight progressively (a method missing in most of today's strength training programs). This was cyclical training in its earliest days, the idea being that as the weight increased the number of reps decreased, and I could get more bang for my buck in terms of strength. But sometimes the weight in hand felt like too much and my body was too tired—or so I thought—to lift more. I remember times when Ralph watched over me while I was doing a set of lifts. As I worked, I started to feel pain taking over, my body aching and screaming for me to stop with the agony already. On top of the screams, there was a cacophony of thoughts overrunning my mind. *Fuck, this is hard. Don't know if I can keep doing this.* With the bar resting on my shoulders as I neared the end of a set of reps, Ralph would say the words, "put your mind to it." I know it's a cliché, but it's like the children's story, *The Little Engine That Could.* As it tried to move up the hill, it repeated "I think I can, I think I can." Ralph inspired the "I think I can" in me, so I tried and I succeeded more times than not.

Ralph wasn't yelling and screaming at me to give it 110 percent or chiding me about being weak, nor was he using some other antiquated coaching rhetoric. He simply asked me to tap in to my grit to overcome the weight of the bar and my self-doubt. Even if I didn't believe I could lift the weight one more time, it was his phrase I surrendered to and believed in. His words showed me that I was more capable than I suspected.

For me, grit was a revolt against the undermining self-talk and mental conditioning I endured much of my life. Ralph was instrumental in showing me that my beliefs were not always as real as I took them to be. Ralph taught me that with enough grit, I could move heavy weights and my body would grow stronger. He made me question myself and my limiting thoughts, and pushed me to consider if I could do more.

GRIT, PAIN, AND ARRIVAL

There's one story during those years with Ralph that I'll never forget. He had this great idea one day—well, great or terrible, depending how you look at it; today, this type of training might not fly. Two of my high school lifting buddies and I, all of us shot-putters and footballers, were lifting one afternoon. I was about seventeen years old. These mates, Bob and Dale, were both a year older than I was and they were very strong dudes, even by today's high standards. Ralph's idea was to pit us against one another in a sort of friendly lifting competition.

Well, little did we know what was coming. We all naively said, "Sure." What a bunch of lemmings we were—no question, we were definitely young and dumb. So Ralph laid out the contest to us. We were going to do three big lifts: the bench press, the squat, and the power clean. With each lift, we'd all do three sets of as many reps as we could, until we failed and couldn't do any more. We'd lift 185 lb. for all three lifts. The goal of the contest was to see who could do the most reps for all nine sets.

The total rep tally grew steadily and I don't think I need to tell you how fatigued we became. Our arm, chest, and shoulder muscles filled with lactic acid. It felt like my muscles had been beaten with a baseball bat. Not only that, but after a while the entire physical system, not just the musculature, began to collapse. Systemic fatigue is just a highfalutin way of describing it; "Fucking-A tired" is what we called it. But all along there was Ralph telling us, "put your mind to it" and "just one more," and just one more we did.

By the end of the three bench-press sets, our rep count was somewhere in the neighborhood of forty-five to sixty. We took a whopping minute to rest, then set up the squat bar at 185 lb. and off we went to the second phase of pain and agony. While the bench press was hard, this would be much harder. Why? Because now we were using the biggest muscles in our bodies and the energy cost for each rep was significantly greater. We were not only squatting our own weight— around 220 lb. at the time for me—but another 185 lb. on top of that. The bench was a lowly warmup lift by comparison. Each set was in the twenty to thirty range, and the last ten reps in each set were taking a full minute at five to six seconds each. But it felt like an eternity. Between reps, I'd try to focus and get enough oxygen, as all of us were panting like we'd run a 400-meter race flat-out. I listened to the indistinct sound of Ralph's voice in the background as my body became more and more numb.

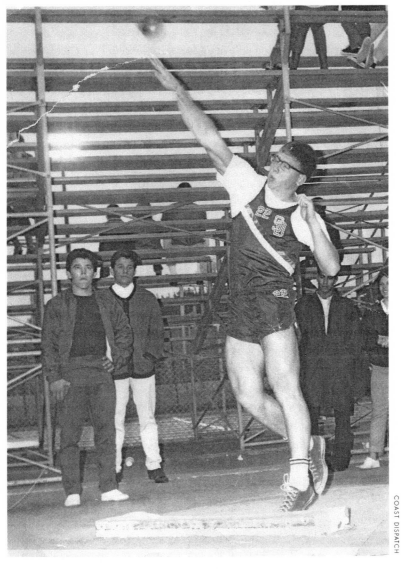

COAST DISPATCH

A boy and his shot, age 16

It's a strange sensation and hard to describe unless you've experienced it, but when adrenaline from physical exertion goes into the system in such huge quantities, it feels like your body almost disappears. For the moment, you're cut off from the pain, though at the same time it's definitely still there. I suppose it's a bit of a fight-or-flight survival mechanism. Whatever it is, I can tell you that the entire body feels disconnected, and the fatigue is so overwhelming that thoughts of whether you're going to survive the pain and suffering dart in and out of consciousness. *Why am I doing this?* was a question that kept popping up in my mind. Ralph knew the answer. At that time, we did not.

Once we'd finished the squat reps, I recall not being able to walk normally. Ralph set up the bar for the power clean, and we all sat quietly in a stupor, waiting to descend into hell again in just a few minutes. The worst part was knowing that the power clean is the most draining and fatiguing of the three lifts: it uses and requires probably 80 percent of your body to lift the weight, plus it's explosive by nature. It has to be explosive in order to get it off the ground and onto your shoulders—it's just wickedly hard. Imagine running the 1500-meter race at the end of the decathlon event, or riding up the infamous Mount Ventoux near the end of the Tour de France. It's harder than hard. We knew that was coming up. The tally for the reps was close, though I was in the lead. I was thinking of survival—not of winning.

Ralph, ever the proctor and wise sage, stood calmly by. He knew that he wasn't pitting us against one another but against ourselves and our own minds. This was a personal test disguised as a competition against buddies. Great coaches and teachers know what the student needs to learn and they will place tasks, in one form or another, in front of their willing disciple to teach what needs to be learned so that the student grows into something she or he didn't even know was possible.

Toward the end of the first set of power cleans, I began to hallucinate, an out-of-body experience where not only was I not in my body but nothing seemed real. Like Alice falling down the rabbit hole, my mind was in an altered state, acting on autopilot. It listened to Ralph and commanded my body to do more, even though it clearly wanted to just fall on the floor in a pool of sweat. But instead I kept pressing on.

By the third and final set, I was still narrowly ahead of Bob and Dale, but I would need to find some magic—or an IV of straight caffeine—to stay in the lead. They were as tenacious of competitors as I've ever come up against. It was during the final set that I placed all my focus on just the next rep. This wasn't preplanned; doing so just happened and it's a visceral memory that lingers in my mind today. There was no thought about the previous rep or how many more I could do; it was just about the present. It became a meditation and all else faded away.

In that last set, I could no longer feel my legs. My back was so tight it felt as though concrete had been poured into my muscles. I could barely take in a breath before I lifted the weight; there was not enough air in the universe to satisfy my heart and muscles. The hallucinations became more frequent as I continued to do just one more rep. The fatigue was indescribable. My body protested, and each thought was a cry of mental anguish.

The final rep came, driven by the last whiff of willpower that I could muster, until I could no longer lift the weight. There was absolutely nothing left. Empty and utterly spent, I sat down and vaguely noticed the pats on my back. I had won. Victory, yes, but it was a costly one. The real "win" was in the mantra given to me that day and that I've used ever since: "put your mind to it." If you put your mind to it, you can do just about anything.

This body numbing event led to epic amounts of soreness and fatigue that lasted a week. Thank god for the healing effects of the saltwater of the nearby Pacific Ocean. Though the experience taught me about my own potential and planted an important seed of knowledge that would continue to grow and flourish over the coming years, it also became apparent that it wasn't to my advantage to go to the punishing levels of maxed-out effort with any regularity.

As a teen, it was a valuable lesson to learn the limits of my body and that I could push beyond pain. But in the three years under Ralph's wing, he only asked us to push to that level once. Once was enough; from that I knew what was possible.

I think of it in the vein of taking out a new Aston Martin on a deserted highway and seeing what it can do in sixth gear. Once you find out what its maximum potential is, it isn't necessarily prudent, useful, or practical to consistently push it to those levels. The thinking is, "Okay, now I know what this baby can do." Maybe there's a day when that knowledge will be useful, although it's hard to imagine why it would be useful other than just for the sheer fun of it. Most of the time the top speed is not useful at all. It's the same with pushing yourself to maximum limits. It might be interesting to see what you can do, but, in the big picture, it is not sensible or helpful for improving consistent performance. More on this in the next chapter.

It wasn't until years later, when I began to recall those sweaty days at the gym, that I realized what Ralph's true gift to me was. His disciplined approach helped me to study myself at a deeper level and explore who I was beyond my self-imposed concepts.

Weightlifting was the context in which Ralph's guidance and mentorship nudged me to understand and harness the power of my mind. Yes, he inspired me to be better, to become stronger, and ultimately to throw the shot put farther, but his primary contribution was to show me that I had the grit to overcome the concepts I defined myself by.

According to Ralph, when in pursuit of a passion or an internal yearning to change and grow, you must create and adhere to a disciplined approach. This idea became my guiding light. Ralph, with his quietude and unbending discipline, inspired me to reach beyond where I already was. He showed me that discipline is a direct reflection of you "gotta wanna": you really, really have to possess the inner drive toward what you're seeking. As the Indian spiritual teacher Nisargadatta Maharaj said in his book *I Am That*, when seeking, "You have to put your mind and your heart on it." Indeed you do.

GAINING GRIT

Own What You Want
Decide what you really want.

To accomplish anything, you must possess the desire to do, achieve, gain, or grow in some way. You "gotta wanna." Without that deep-seated desire, the will to take action will dissipate into indifference.

Your desire can relate to anything—taking on an event, making a change in your physical and mental well-being, learning something new. It doesn't matter what it is, but you have to want it. Here, it's the wanting that's important. Oftentimes, fear—whether recognized as such or not—can be so intense that it inhibits desire. When you're afraid, you might think to yourself, *Why bother wanting anything, when I know I'm not going to get it anyway?* But in order to move forward, facing that fear of failure is key to making it to the starting point.

Having a goal comes with the possibility of disappointment. Like novelist Richard Yates said, "If you don't try anything, you can't fail... It takes back bone to lead the life you want." That's grit right there—wanting something while knowing that you might not get it. But one thing I can guarantee is that you *definitely* won't get it if you don't want it first.

> *Is there something in your life that you've always wanted, but been afraid to pursue?*
> *Has fear—of discomfort, the unknown, failure—stopped you from trying something new?*
> *Have you avoided challenges and set limits on yourself based on old information?*

If you answered yes to any of these questions, then it may be time to examine your self-imposed edge and go for something that will make you test it.

DO A REALITY CHECK

Once you set your sights on something, there's one question you need to ask yourself: How will this goal make your life better? Consider the value it will ultimately bring to your physical, mental, or emotional growth, to your health and generally feeling of awesomeness. Will it add to it or subtract?

For instance, I wouldn't talk you out of an attempt to break the world record in eating sixty-seven hot dogs in eight minutes, but it might be prudent to question what that goal will do for you other than extending your stomach lining like a helium balloon and causing you to feel awful. Yeah, you may break the record, but that requires a lot of suffering just to say you did it and get a few likes on Facebook. Just saying. It's your choice, but be clear on the effects and the value of getting there and fulfilling that desire.

For an example that might be a little closer to home: let's say you're having a mid-life moment and your inner critic is saying, *Geez, I'm in the worst shape of my life. I need to get my ass back in gear before the damage is permanent.* Right in time, you hear that some buddies are planning to run a half marathon, so you decide to opt in and join them. You've found a way to get fit (and ultimately, feel more confident) again. And, when you assess the accessibility of this challenge, you determine that it's going to be hard as hell but you have the time, energy, and desire to make it happen. That's just great—I love the idea of taking on some sort of physical feat that can test your grit while giving you something that is worthwhile in the long term.

A reality check isn't just about questioning your ultimate gains, it's also about examining the costs. Since there's a cost incurred by pursuing any goal, it's best to know what the cost/reward ratio is for you before you fully commit yourself. It's a simple equation. Assuming you have a finite amount of time, energy, and money, how much is your goal going to set you back? Being honest with yourself—and not tricking yourself with your own personal variation of BS—will help you determine whether you'll actually follow through. Many a great intention has fizzled because of an unrealistic view of the total cost and the downstream consequence of a big decision.

Are you willing to do what it takes?

What impact will this goal have on your daily life, including work, family, and friends?

What are you willing to sacrifice to achieve this goal?
Are you being realistic in terms of time and energy required?

STAY THE COURSE

When your journey begins, you will probably be trying new things. It will be exciting at first, and you'll be riding high on the newness of it all. But at the same time, you'll likely be forced to confront the same old habits, patterns, and beliefs that you've encountered before. No worries. Just hang in there—use your grit and know that being able to recognize these old patterns as they arise is critical to moving forward. Practice being aware of where your doubts tend to lurk. We all have internal hecklers, and perhaps you recognize these kinds of thoughts:

I don't have enough time to . . .
I would but I'm not good enough to . . .
I don't think I can because . . .
I'm not smart enough to . . .
I'm not strong enough to . . .

There are many more that you'll encounter along the path to your desired goal. Fear not. Just don't reward such doubts with attention. Simply watch them and do not fight them. Maintain your earnest resolve as they come and go. The more you engage with doubt, the more entangled with it you'll become. The power it has over you is in direct proportion to your investment in it. Though these heckler thoughts may seem real, they are just ghosts until we give them life.

PUT YOUR MIND TO IT

Now it's time to take action and go, go, go by "putting your mind to it." Think of these words as being the spark to rev the engine of your grit.

There are many challenges in life. Walking the path of self-improvement is no exception. But once you begin to see the results of your efforts, you can draw on the memory of those experiences in the future when you feel yourself flagging. If you don't face new challenges, you won't increase your grit. The mantras that I use to call upon grit is Ralph's "put your mind to it" and *"I can do it."*

Remember the part toward the end of the movie *Top Gun* where Maverick is in a dogfight with the Russians? Mav's copilot and fellow fighter pilots are yelling and screaming at him to engage the MIG fighter in his sights, but he's lost in the memories of mistakenly engaging a friendly pilot in the past, leading to the death of his copilot, Goose. With fear and doubt overwhelming him, he isn't able to pull the trigger. He's stuck in the past and can't engage with what's in front of him. Then, finally, something shifts in him, and the badass Maverick spurns the memory of failure and does what he needs to do. The hero emerges again and defeats the foe of his mind along with the MIGs.

Most of us are like Maverick. Life gets tough. Grit carries us through. "I can do it" keeps us on track. And sometimes a teacher can help get you there faster.

FIND A YODA

A gifted teacher or mentor can expedite your journey toward your goal. It's his or her gift of awareness that helps you see what you don't or can't on your own. The value of having a good teacher is that he or she can help you understand where your thinking is misaligned with your goal, and where you're causing suffering—thereby accelerating the speed of your progress.

Luke Skywalker from *Star Wars* famously had Yoda, who taught him the ways of "the force" and how to harness it. Neo from *The Matrix* had Morpheus and the Oracle to show him how to see reality for what it was.

If you seek a teacher, look for someone who can listen to you and, better yet, ask you questions—even the really hard ones. (Your best teacher will not always tell you what you want to hear.) S/he needs to know you at the level where s/he can see your underlying assumptions and help you correct your course when you are veering away from it. So it's critical that you are honest and open, and that you let your teacher observe all sides of you so that s/he *can* see.

A teacher should be curious about what makes you tick. S/he should be able to push you beyond your self-imposed concepts and also be able to hold you back when you're not physically, mentally, or emotionally ready for the next step. Of course, sometimes working with a teacher can initially be frustrating or uncomfortable. This might be a sign of a good teacher—he or she is pushing all your buttons, and in the moment that sucks. But even if you feel resistance—or like you're spinning your wheels—later on you might see why the teacher taught in that way. This is a long-game situation, and it could take a little while to get that perspective. But like everything, the path is not always direct or linear. There's a cycle to building momentum: failure informs success just as much as success informs failure. This is probably not clear now, but don't worry—we'll get into it in the next chapter.

YOU CAN—WITH GRIT

We all have the ability to push beyond our expectations when we access our grit—one time, and many times. Filling your reservoir of grit comes from the small steps of practice, and seeing what's possible through this practice. Grit is essential for moving you toward your ambitions and desires, but heed one lesson I learned through my own mistakes: Don't become addicted to using the extreme side of this acquired power as a way of living life; instead, tap into it wisely, as needed, and for the purpose of breaking the bonds of self-limiting thinking. Though the Aston Martin can travel at 170 mph, that's just not a sustainable pace. Stopping now and then to view the vistas while appreciating the distance you've already traveled will help you value the experience of meeting your goal, not just the thrill of crossing the finish line. This is balance.

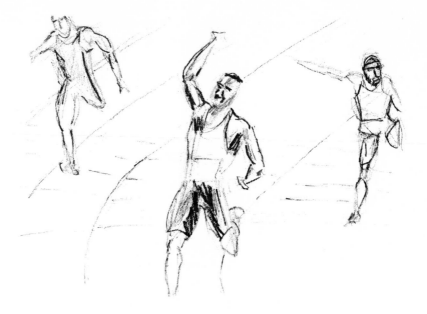

Patience is also a form of action.

AUGUSTE RODIN

LESS IS MORE

Just when you're sure you've got it all figured out, something comes along that tips your world sideways. This something might make you lose your footing, but don't immediately jump to believing it's a bad development. In fact, it could bring an "aha" moment that fundamentally changes the way you think and behave—for the better.

Let's put it this way: sometimes in life, just when you think you need to go south to reach your goal, the next lesson points you north. Go there.

Coming into contact with a new—and therefore, threatening—idea forces us to examine ourselves, and for most of us, that's a real uncomfortable situation. We might have to admit that we aren't as smart as we thought we were. Think of all those folks who railed against the idea that the world doesn't revolve around the sun. Can you think of anything more threatening than the suggestion that we aren't, in fact, the center of the universe? But if we are truly invested in learning and improving, getting to that moment of discomfort and seeing it through is when some big changes start to happen.

As I reflect back on my time under the guidance of the great track and field coach Bill Bowerman at the University of Oregon, I realize that his teachings wove their way through the rest of my athletic career and beyond. Bill was a great teacher, a gifted tactician, and a sly jokester who made his athletes laugh at themselves even as he pushed their boundaries. Even better, he went out on a limb, teaching techniques that were contrary to the conventional wisdom of the time. He was one of the teachers who, as soon as I thought I knew the best way to improve myself and my performance, would show me there was still more to learn; sometimes the new lessons ended up contradicting the old ones in one way or another.

This did not mean that the old lessons were not "true"; instead, I had to face the idea that there are more sides to the "truth" than I had previously imagined.

After my time playing high school football and weight lifting with Ralph Kroger, I thought that in order to succeed, I needed to push hard and harder still—100 percent wasn't good enough, I had to give 110. This line of thinking gave me such a narrow range of options— only one, actually: go hard or go home. Most people have this same all-or-nothing philosophy, that if you don't push yourself to the max, it isn't worth your time. This is the hernia method: push until you lose your guts.

Fortunately, since I seem to have a knack for meeting great teachers at the right moment, I came across the idea of "less is more." And this, my friends, is probably what got me to the Olympics. The belief that you can gain more by doing less goes against the grain, the cultural myths about the path to success. Discovering that I could reach my goals using less energy and having less mental strife was a huge change in my thinking.

This chapter is about that profound lesson, that less can be more. While Ralph Kroger taught me to push it to the limit every now and then, just to test myself and my limiting beliefs, Bill Bowerman taught patience and moderation. Bill's teaching was ahead of its time, and it truly was a great gift.

AWAKENING TO LESS IS MORE WITH BILL BOWERMAN

I went to the University of Oregon from 1968 to 1972. *Go Ducks!* Bill Bowerman's last four years of coaching happened to align with those early years of my training—great timing and very lucky for me. He has a few claims to fame: he invented the Nike shoe, served as head coach of the 1972 Olympic US Track and Field team, and he was the man behind many world record holders, Olympic medalists, and collegiate champions. He was larger than life, and one of the greatest track and field coaches in the history of the sport.

When I first arrived at U of O, my training on the track and in the weight room hadn't changed much from my high school days. Whether I was doing deadlifts or throwing a shot put, I pushed it hard almost every day. The only difference was that now after my "binges" of pushing myself to the brink of exhaustion, I would often get sick.

During my first two years in college, I suffered from multiple terrible sinus infections, needing massive amounts of antibiotics to kill off the invading bacteria. My poor immune system was traumatized from overtraining, but if I didn't go further each and every practice, I'd get seriously pissed off, ranting and raving and throwing epic tantrums during which the assistant coaches would slowly back away, putting distance between themselves and me, the red hot volcano. Over time, these episodes became less forceful and less frequent, mostly because of Bill's influence.

During my freshman year, Bill came by the practice ring, where we threw our 16 lb. steel balls once or twice a week. He usually coached me on how to improve my technique and how to be more efficient. He talked about my position in the ring, my posture, and the height of the throw at release. The whole time, he didn't say a single word about trying to throw farther. *Is this guy for real?* I wondered incredulously.

What I didn't realize then was that his focus on technique and timing was a way to get me to focus on the work itself, rather than using all of my energy in *trying.* So, I worked on my technique—timing, position, finding a rhythm— and discovered new ways to encourage my body to relax. He was creating the ethos that quality was more important than quantity. This was, to say the least, a different tack than what I was used to, and counterintuitive to my notions of performance training. Nobody liked to go all out and test the limits more than I did, and initially this training frustrated the hell out of me. But my body—and my frequent sinus infections—were telling me something, and thanks to Bill, I began to listen.

The next eye-opening chapter with Bill was a series of practice sessions with him and a guy named Neal Steinhauer. I won't forget those sessions as long as I live. Neal was six years my senior and a former University of Oregon Duck. At the time, Neal held the world record for the indoor shot put event with a throw of 68'11". As a sophomore, I was lucky enough to room with Neal while he was in the vortex of making a comeback, trying to make the Olympic team in 1972, a couple of years away.

OK, so I was this twenty-year-old who'd thrown maybe 60', and I was still really low on the totem pole of American throwers. So when Bill asked me to join him and Neal for some intimate throwing sessions, I was stoked, just electrified with adrenaline. Throwing with one of the greatest throwers, and in front of one of the greatest coaches in track and field, was an incredible opportunity.

The training sessions were held in what was called the "bubble"—an air-filled field house about 75 meters long, inflated during the wet and windy season to give a us a little relief from the elements. The air was maybe three degrees warmer inside than out, so it wasn't exactly what I would call warm during those long gray Oregon winters. But I didn't really even notice it then—I was buff and tough and impervious to all but the moment. During these sessions, the world seemed very small: it was only Bill, Neal, and me. Nothing else existed.

Bill instructed us to take three throws in a row. Our first throw was intended to be easy, with almost no effort. We were to just use our bodies—not our arms—for the final part of the throw. For me, though, this wasn't easy. The second throw was to be of medium effort with complete follow through, using the arms in a relaxed, fluid throw. The goal wasn't to throw far but to find a rhythm and to make it feel easy. The last throw was hard: we were to put a lot of effort into it, but at the same time maintain the technique and the rhythm of the previous two throws. If all the timing, fluidity, and ease went out the window on this final throw, then the exercise wasn't considered successful. No grunting, just grace. We were to put forth the effort but not make it look or feel effortful. We were trying not to try.

As excited as I was to be working with Bill, I was also skeptical, thinking that the exercise would be a waste of time. I just didn't understand how this was going to be beneficial—it was so against what I thought was the right way. By that point, I had gotten so used to tension, seriousness, and the rush of adrenalin that an easy throw seemed less than worthless. *What's the point?* I thought. Needless to say, it took a while for me to fully embrace his ideology.

Slowly as a glacier moves, I started to get it. Those hard throws began to feel less tension-filled, more relaxed. As days turned into months, the gradual realization that this way of training was both easier

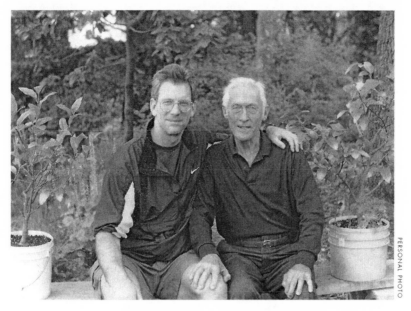

Bill Bowerman and me, circa 1997

and more efficient culminated in an epic "aha" moment. I started to see that it didn't have to be hard to be good—just the opposite. I found a rhythm and an ease in the movement, so even with buckets of adrenaline and mountains of desire behind the effort, I could hold my drive at bay and make real progress. I opened up to a new "truth," that less is more.

Bill gave me a rude awakening that I didn't want but definitely needed. Talk about making a foundational shift.

THE MESSAGE

I wasn't the first athlete to have my foundation rocked by Bill's advice. Bill had also worked with an up-and-coming long-distance runner at the University of Oregon named Kenny Moore. Kenny's plan to get himself to the next level was to increase his mileage to over 100 miles a week, as that was what others around the country were doing. Bill pointed out, most bluntly I'm sure, that Kenny had been sick and injured quite a bit in the past year. Bill challenged Kenny, asking him why he thought that he should run even more miles. "Do you want to do mindless work," Bill asked him, "or do you want to improve?" Boom. Kenny got the blunt message. He went on to run the marathon in the Olympics, finishing 4th place in 1968 games in Munich a few years later. Bill's words of wisdom paid off for Kenny.

It's amusing and a bit of a conundrum that the company Bowerman co-founded, Nike, coined the tagline "Just do it." While we do have to just do it, Bill taught us *how* to do it by "training not straining" as he wrote in his book, *Jogging*. He deemed rest to be as important as training, and held that both were essential to progress.

Because of this, the athletes on my team were rarely injured. Runners who were not making progress in competition or who often got sick were told in no uncertain terms that they better not be seen taking early morning "easy" runs. Though these runs were only three to six miles with very low intensity, if a runner was showing signs of overtraining, Bowerman would forbid him from heading out for a run in the damp Eugene air. Instead, he'd order the runner to sleep in and let his body fully recover.

When you have a bunch of testosterone-filled athletes with Type A personalities, it takes a tough, wise coach with a sense of the overall game plan to implement a style of training that might challenge their ways of thinking. Bill already knew what we needed to know: *that sheer will is a sometimes wonderful and sometimes terrible force.* Most of us were slaves to our wills and quite unskilled at truly listening to our bodies. Bill forced us to question our mindsets, pay attention to our bodies, and take time off when needed. It was tough love at its best. And we benefited greatly because of it.

Though it took a while for Bill's teachings to get through my thick skull, I eventually came around. As the saying goes, "the proof is in the pudding," and my pudding was that each year I improved substantially. Coming into my freshman year, my best throw was 53'. After the first year that I worked with Bill, I improved my best mark by six feet, which was huge, something like 10 percent better than the previous year. By the time I left U of O, my best throw was 66'4"—the second farthest throw of any Oregon Duck. Bill Bowerman showed me the way.

HOW TO GET MORE BY DOING LESS
Reel It In—Pain Doesn't Equal Gain

Discomfort, effort, sweat, and a few tears are just fine—in moderation. But working to the point of pain and exhaustion consistently and often is a surefire way to get hurt, sick, or worse.

The conventional wisdom of the day is go faster, go harder, work until you can't work no more. It's an all-or-nothing mentality, and it disconnects people from their bodies. The Statue of Liberty might as well read *no pain, no gain* to welcome newcomers to US soil. Americans are known for their long work hours, lack of vacation time, and sedentary lifestyles. We seem to be getting chubbier and more frazzled all the time. We tend to live in extremes—devoting ourselves to work at the cost of our bodies; then, as we realize that our bodies are falling apart, getting into the latest and greatest high-intensity workout craze that often leads to injury, fatigue, or burnout. Plus, throughout it all, we continue to feel a general sense of anxiety from the constant worry that we're never doing enough. Everything is supposed to be so damn hard core. Why? Because we're a Puritan land, and we have to have a rigid and harsh work ethic to be good.

Whether you're a high-level athlete training for your next championship or a desk jockey who wants to look good in a bathing suit, just chill out. A myopic vision of health and fitness will thwart long term success.

What are your notions around *no pain, no gain?*

Change it Up...Consistently

The earliest Olympic athletes used a sophisticated system called "the tetras." This was a four-day system with varied effort levels. The first day was the preparation day, with high intensity and short duration. The second day was a day of intensity; it was both strenuous and of long duration. The third day was the day of rest, when athletes would do very light activities or just take the day off. The fourth day was a medium intensity day, with relatively strenuous activities. In those ancient times, athletes varied the structure and intensity of their training to maximize results.

You too will greatly benefit by approaching a practice in this way, by acknowledging that your physical energy and mental state are constantly shifting, and by matching your effort to your condition. When you recognize that each of the four effort levels is valuable, deciding how—or whether—to exercise at the gym, hike up a mountain, meet a deadline, or take a sick day becomes a whole lot easier.

Workout intensity can be divided into four levels: zilch, easy, medium, and hard. All of these levels are important for sustainable training. Use the following effort-level scale to help you organize your workouts and structure your time.

Zilch:
0% effort.
Just plain old resting, necessary for recovery.

Easy:
10–30 % effort.
A good starting point when getting back into exercising; a range for activity when movement is desired but energy is low; a range to train on off-days.

Medium:
40–60 % effort.
More exertion, while being manageable for long durations.

Hard:
70–90 % effort.
Nearing maximum effort, usually for short durations.

If you're not totally sure what each of these levels feels like, try this experiment. Learning how to identify your version of easy, medium, and hard (and zilch) will help you organize your practice.

1.   Walk or run as slowly as you can. And I mean SLOW. As in, a turtle could kick your ass if this was a race. In theory, you could do this all day. Start at 10 percent, and over the next couple of minutes, slowly amp up the effort level to 30 percent.

2. Increase your effort another 10 percent. Now you're moving from "easy" to "medium." You should now be experiencing a palpable level of effort. Heart rate and breathing rate has increased. Continue until you reach about 60 percent.

3. Increase your effort another 10 percent. Now you're moving into "hard," and you're working hard and breathing hard. Perhaps you're getting tired. Make sure that this is your version of hard. Be careful and only push yourself in a way that's safe.

4. If you're up for it, kick it up one more notch and add another 10–20 percent. Take it to your max, then stop and rest.

The purpose of this experiment is to experience what your body feels like at each level and to be able to—with practice—choose what level is best suited for an activity on any given day.

Familiarity with different levels of effort isn't just useful in the world of exercise, by the way—it can also be helpful for other parts of your life. For instance, there are days when you're tired, and cleaning the house from top to bottom will only make you more tired (and maybe a little grumpy, too). There are days at the office when you feel on top of your game, and it makes sense to use that to your advantage and finally get to all those stacks on your desk. Being able to tell when and how much effort is needed can help you to use your energy in a more efficient and productive way.

Follow the 80 Percent Rule

Getting the opportunity to watch the best athletes train, to be exposed to the knowledge of some of the world's greatest coaches, and to experiment on my own, I've come to believe that the hardest you need to push yourself on a "hard day" is about 80 percent of your maximum. This is plenty for the layperson. For a seasoned high-level athlete with years of slow progressive training experience, the range can go up to 90 percent. However, going to this point is rarely needed. Usually, the athlete will save that maximum push for competition.

Sure, we have to push ourselves to the max occasionally to see what we're made of, but the more we do it, the more recovery the body needs. You don't have to push it to the limit to develop physical strength and an elevated fitness level. Working at 80 percent allows you to maintain your energy reserves, to recover quickly, and to come back the next day without feeling debilitated.

The 3 REs: REgenerate, REcapture, REvitalize

If you've ever used an epoxy glue, you know that it's made of two resins that, when added together, create the magical substance that binds. The super strong bond is created only when those two resins are mixed in equal amounts; if you use just one to fix that busted dish or reattach that table leg, you will end up with a broken dish and a three-legged table. It takes both parts; neither one is more or less important than the other.

Rest and physical effort are the two compounds that make up a healthy lifestyle. By incorporating both into your activities in equal measure, you will recover quickly and have the energy to face life's challenges. You'll get sick less often, your energy will be higher and more consistent, and you'll just feel better. It's all about maintaining homeostasis—when the body is out of balance, then rest, recovery, healthy eating, lots of sleeping, and other methods of caretaking help bring the body back into equilibrium.

If you think I'm living in a *la-la* land where everyone exercises all the time, don't worry, I'm not. I see very clearly that for many Americans, too much rest is the problem. Their routine is: sit in front of a screen, eat fast food, repeat. Overexertion isn't their problem, just the opposite. The body doesn't work so well if it's not getting time to move, and half of the *yin-yang* is missing.

But I do also see a lot of people who fall into the other extreme. If you're anything like me, you lean toward the side of overtraining, overworking, over pushing. Rest, recovery, and doing less is your missing ingredient.

So do something nice and easy for yourself, something fun that doesn't have *being productive* as the end goal. Go for a walk, get a massage, take a sauna, read a book. Turn off the phone and computer. Trust me, you'll feel better later.

Finding Less—Moving, Performing, and Living Better

I understood what Bowerman meant all those years ago, but as I've thought about the wisdom of his coaching since then, I have truly come to appreciate what he was advising: patience and moderation leads to sustainable results. Most of us want what we want, and we want it now. Often we believe that we'll get what we want more quickly if we work harder, stronger, and faster, grunting and sweating every step of the way. But that method comes with a price: namely injury, fatigue, stress and strain, and, ultimately, the creation of patterns that are unsustainable and self-defeating. Plus it's not fun. Steady progress or maintenance over a lifetime is the real goal, and practicing moderation by way of easy, medium, hard, and zilch is the means to do that.

No matter what you are trying to accomplish, you need to consider the easiest way to get there. I've known many people—from desk jockeys to Olympic athletes—who have burned out through overtraining or overworking and not taking time to recover. Bowerman would be all over those people. The people who recognize that they don't need to do it all, do it hardest, and do it best all of the time usually find that they have more energy to figure out what actually needs to be done, and ultimately they lead happier, healthier lives.

So don't be your own worst enemy. When you're feeling the itch to strain and strive or add one more thing to your to-do list, ask yourself this: Do I really need to do this? What is the greatest reward for the least cost? What is the least amount of energy I need to exert to make true progress? Questioning yourself may be hard, but it's worth it. There are many great teachers out there, including you. You just gotta be open to the lesson—and to not making everything so damn hard all the time when it could just as easily be easy.

You can only train as hard as you can recover.
APOLO OHNO, EIGHT-TIME OLYMPIC MEDALIST
IN SHORT TRACK SPEED SKATING

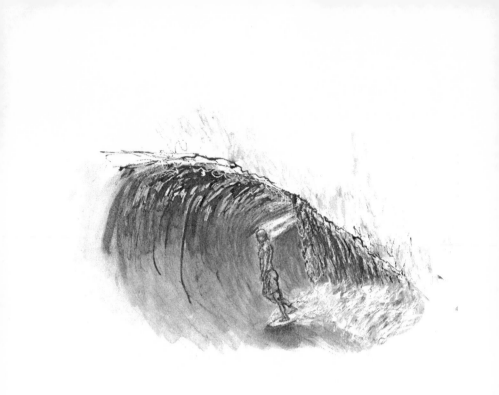

You must shift your sail with the wind

ITALIAN PROVERB

MOVING WITH THE CYCLES

When you slow down and take a look around, you'll notice this clear and simple phenomenon: everywhere, at all times and in all stages, cycles are happening. The most obvious and most confounding one is the life cycle, from birth to death—no escaping that one. Everything has a birth and a death, from the fruit fly to the Milky Way, and everything is in constant flux, succumbing to chaos and then reorganizing itself only to succumb again.

We've all experienced the cycles of nature: the changing of the seasons, the trees shedding their leaves and the birds making their yearly trek to warmer climates. There are fluctuations in the tides, turns in the economy, shift from feast to famine, the waxing and waning of the moon. We can get real macro here, all the way on up to the fact that someday our galaxy will die and the billions of years of the earth's life—not to mention the puny decades of our own individual lives—will be as quickly forgotten in the blink of an eye. But let's keep it simple; let's talk about us.

Our bodies will inform us about a variety of cycles. From external cues from the environment, we make decisions every day. Sometimes we don sweaters and sometimes we wear bathing suits, without really having to ask ourselves which is the better choice. We naturally adapt and adjust (albeit begrudgingly at times) in order to avoid suffering.

And, at the same time, there are the constant internal fluctuations that both motivate and result from behavior: the waking and the sleeping, the hunger and the satiation, the drive for sex and the drive for a hot shower. First we're hungry, then we're satisfied, then we're hungry again. The broader environment has an influence—heavy, warm pasta meal in the winter, anyone?—and at the same time every individual cell has its own needs, its own cycles. Our body speaks, and sometimes we listen. When we don't listen, the body will make us pay attention eventually. Every moment within these cycles both leads to and is completely entrenched in the next.

Every day, the human body goes through a circadian cycle. Its fluctuations are made up of biochemical, physiological, and behavioral cycles that are both emerging from within the organism and simultaneously influenced by the environment. Every twenty-four hours or so, we humans go through shifts in sleep, hormone levels, temperature, and so on. For the most part, we don't have to pay attention to this cycle—it sort of just manages itself (that is, until you try to work the graveyard shift or down a bowl of ice-cold gazpacho in the dead of winter).

When you have a body, there are two cycles that are important to be aware of—the shorter ones occurring hour to hour and day to day, and the longer ones that span months, years, an entire lifetime. Every day, cycles in our energy shift. Some days we feel like we "got it" and some days we don't, no matter how much coffee we've consumed. We are subject to varying waves of internal energy that can be affected by numerous factors: food, sleep, emotions, stress, mental habits, physical activity, genetic predisposition, and age.

Meanwhile, the longer cycles happen more slowly and with more subtlety, and they require awareness to adjust and adapt our overall game plan. As we age, our needs and wants will also change along with our bodies and circumstances, and they require acceptance and flexible evolution in order to keep as healthy as possible.

For example, many of us like to run to stay fit. But I've noticed after many years of training that there often comes a day when a runner gets hurt—tears an ACL, fractures a foot—and an immediate change to accommodate is required. This is sometimes just a momentary change in a cycle, but it could also be an ending. Now, the runner can no longer pound the pavement in the way that she or he has gotten used to. This can be really difficult emotionally and physically; it can feel like a big loss. But, the body is the boss, and as much as the ex-runner wants to be in control, it just ain't gonna happen. When this happens to you, you *have* to go with what's happening—you don't really have a choice—no matter how much it sucks. So you make some changes. You buy a bike, a helmet, a spandex biking outfit, grab some new buddies to ride with, and a new phase begins. Or you grab a headband and a mat and take up Jazzercise. Whatever you do, you've adapted—you've dealt with the inevitable changes and kept your cool. And, eventually, if you're lucky enough to live a good long time, you'll still be moving, but it's likely that your activities will get gentler and gentler as you go. And that's just fine.

If you're like me, you may want the fun phases of the cycle—the times of good health, financial success, or professional achievement— to last forever. The more unpalatable times—the long period of recovery after injury, an economic downswing, an enduring personal hardship—are ones most of us want to escape from or avoid. But, regardless of our individual desires or aversions, there are cycles within everything, and nothing stays the same, so it's up to us to deal with it and to make the most of that over which we have so little control.

It's truly fascinating to observe the reactions we have to the cycles. Increased awareness and the practice of acceptance can help us to be more equipped to choose how to react. Of course, most of us want to walk the straight and narrow; we want life to be organized and sensible. So what do we do when something comes along that blocks our path or knocks us off center? What do we do when chaos disrupts our calm? What it comes down to is this: you can either flow with the changes of life or against them. Ultimately, you do have a choice in this, and you retain a little sliver of power within the forces of change that are so much bigger and stronger than you are. Choosing to flow with them might just make life a little easier; going against them is like refusing to change out of your bathing suit when summer comes to an end—all you'll get is frostbite for your efforts. The seasons don't care what you want.

The body knows what it needs, and if you don't pay attention, it'll *make* you pay attention. Now we've all heard the phrase "listen to your body" or "pay attention" a thousand and one times. It's a very useful reminder, but at this point it may have lost its punch. If that's the case, adding an expletive can go a long way in cranking things up, which is why I like to say: pay fucking attention!

When you strain your shoulder on game day, it's generally going to be better for you if you stay home with a pack of ice and a hot water bottle instead of trying to play it out. You can always choose to play through the pain, and if you're a twenty-two-year-old professional football player, your ability to heal quickly can make it possible and that $5 million contract can make it worth it. But if you're a sixty-two-year-old professional accountant, relaxing into the healing process and letting your body take its slow but steady course will probably be your best option. You can also choose to fight it till the cows come home, but all you'll be doing is wasting your time and energy, making yourself grumpy, and aggravating an injury instead of healing it, when you could be giving yourself a much-needed break instead.

What I'm really talking about is knowing when, within a cycle, hard work will be productive and when letting go is the best choice: to observe what's really happening, and adapting to that rather than fooling yourself into believing that your agenda and your will is going to trump reality; to choose a way of being that is fluid and harmonious. This is the ultimate success. Being observant of what's happening within the cycle will help you find an easier, more fluid way, and will promote a more harmonious, softer life.

In the first chapter, we talked about going to the max, and in the previous chapter, we talked about doing less. I hope you see from this chapter the necessity of both, of flowing with the physical and nonphysical cycles of your life. This is a how-to guide to move with and not against the day-to-day cycles of your energy and the longer cycles of aging, and how to gracefully modify your game plan to help you feel good, perform optimally, live the best life possible—with less effort and greater ease.

A CHANGE IN PLAN, A CYCLE ENDED

I graduated from the University of Oregon in the spring of 1973. It took me a year longer than most because I had no clue what I wanted my major to be. At the end of my senior year in 1972, for the first time I thought about what I wanted to get out of college other than an unofficial degree in shot putting and beer consumption. At that moment, a brilliant idea crossed my mind: I would become a doctor. So off I went to sign up for all the prerequisite classes for pre-med. After two quarters of Ds and Cs in classes like physics and organic chemistry (I performed much more admirably in jewelry making, philosophy, and PE), I began to sense that this might not work out as planned. And on top of that, I absolutely hated it. Call me crazy, but I've come to believe that hating an activity is generally a subtle clue that maybe it's time to do something else.

I went to see a counselor, and I asked her, "With all the classes I've taken, what degree am I closest to?" Lucky for me, a general social science degree was in my grasp and only a couple of classes away. Bingo; I graduated.

My first foray into the working world beyond athletics was at a local Eugene law office, where I was a clerk. I had no idea what the hell I was doing, but fortunately my boss was a patient teacher. Sitting long hours doing research, serving subpoenas, and wading through books that weighed almost as much as my shot put was hard for me. I wasn't used to all that sedentariness. I found that the more I sat around, the more tired I got. Though I tackled the jobs he gave me and even managed to not create any extra lawsuits, I knew this just wasn't happening for me in the long-term.

Meanwhile, I had pretty much taken an entire year off from training. On the side, I was making a few bucks as a graduate assistant track coach for Bill, coaching a couple of moderately talented throwers. For me, this was way more fun than the law office gig, plus I seemed to have a knack for it. Out on the field with those guys was where I learned how to be a teacher (and maybe even how to be a B-level psychologist).

By then it was the summer of 1973. And I was still asking myself, *Now what am I going to do?*

The next Olympic Games were two-and-a-half years away, and since I had nothing else lined up, I thought, *What the hell. Why not give it a shot and see if I can make the team?* Looking back, this seems like such naiveté. Sort of like, *Yeah, I'm just going to go down to the mini mart and see if I can buy a winning lottery ticket.* Glad I didn't over-think it too much back then.

With this new goal in mind, I packed my VW blue-and-white two-tone bus—with self-made bed, hippie-designer fabric curtains, and all my meager belongings—and rocking the cool leather visor, I hit the highway to San Jose, California, 550 long miles south of Eugene.

San Jose was attracting a mass of great athletes from around the country because of its good weather, good training facilities, and a general vibe that was starting to build there. I too wanted to find out what was "happening" at the Woodstock of track and field. There I found a bunch of experienced veteran athletes as well as the next generation of elite track athletes, many of whom were seeking the same brass ring that I was. We were all vying to make it to the top three of the 1976 Olympic Trials, thereby winning a spot on the US Olympic team.

I found a cheap apartment, one of those monstrous three-acre maze-like compounds with a bazillion small pools, and I started working as a waiter at The Garrett, a restaurant specializing in fondue, fancy meat and cheese plates, foo-foo sandwiches, and sangria for the people of the Los Gatos, Saratoga, and San Jose areas. The tips I made, plus the hundreds of dollars' worth of food I ate on shift each night (slightly more than the allotment of one meal per night per employee), gave me the freedom to train during the day. It was a simple, easy life for a young man on his own, and to this day I have some nostalgia for those times.

While training at the San Jose State track facilities, I befriended Al Feuerbach, then the world record holder in the shot put event. Caitlyn Jenner (formerly Bruce Jenner) trained there too, as did many other would-be Olympians. In fact, thirteen athletes from various sports who trained in that area made the 1976 Olympic team. We worked off one another's intensity and energy, which pulled us all up beyond what we could have done on our own. Slowly I became one of the guys, accepted as a sincere seeker of the prize: making the team. We were friendly, but at the same time we knew that ultimately we were in competition, vying for the same three spots on the podium. We were wary of getting too close.

Usually, all of us practiced our individual events at the track complex and then congregated at the local YMCA, which was the weight-lifting haven for all the athletes, not just those in track and field. The Saturday afternoon lifting sessions were like a Debutantes' Ball. It was the place to see and be seen, to show your stuff. We lifted huge weights and later gossiped about who did what and with how much effort. We were like a little family, living in our own little world.

After watching Al perform his daily ritual of warming up, training, and throwing over the course of the first half year, I felt a light go on in my head. The light involved some simple observations and questions: Al is smaller than I am. I'm a few percentage points stronger than he is. His technique is more fluid and snappy, but all totaled up it doesn't equate—I shouldn't be five feet behind him. Why can't I throw farther?

As I looked back on the last bit of time, I realized that I hadn't made any great gains. I had thrown 66'5" as my best in college, but now my throwing was stagnant—no improvement in almost two years. Not only was I not making progress, I was also feeling a lot of tension in my body and I just wasn't having as much fun as I used to.

That's when it started to dawn on me that something was off, that I was missing something or not utilizing something…I didn't know what it was but I knew that if I didn't figure it out soon, the next two years would fly by and I'd have no chance of reaching my goal. I needed a big improvement and needed it pronto. By observing Al, I was going to be able to see my weaknesses as reflected in his strengths, and this was going to help me change.

ONE CYCLE ENDS AND ANOTHER BEGINS

As I intently watched Al warm up and stretch for an hour or so before his training began, my perspective shifted. His warmup differed greatly from my warmup, which was usually very short—more like a quick, impatient nod to warming up than actually giving myself time to stretch and focus. From his longer session, he achieved a looseness and suppleness in his body, and I began to deduce that this was a big factor in the fluidity and ease of his throws. They just looked effortless, like he was a dancer moving through the seven-foot metal ring.

So, with this new point of view, I had a new choice. I could either continue training the same way I had been, or I could take a new direction. I opted for the latter. With that decision, one cycle had come to an end and a new cycle had begun.

35

I started buying illustrated books on yogasana, or yoga poses. I began a morning regimen of stretching—what I call mobilizing. Attired with layers of T-shirts, close-fitting training suits, and a top layer of loose-fitting cotton sweat pants and tops, I would slowly begin what would be my first workout of the day. The sessions usually lasted forty-five minutes to an hour, and by the end I'd have sweated through the first two layers of clothing. I had created my own hot yoga.

Along with using the instructions from the yoga books, I created my own movements and positions that I instinctually knew would counter the tightness made by years of training. As I was mobilizing, I noticed that when I pushed too hard, my body would freeze. I was often tempted to push, since that was my baseline belief about training, but whenever I did that the tension grew instead of diminished. This led to a bodily awareness and an ability to discern between different states at a more subtle level. I was opening and softening through these movements and undoing what took years to create, while also simply learning about my body and how it worked.

My mental focus during the body-bending sessions was the exhalation, deep and long with each breath. My mind would wander, and refocusing on the breath would pull me back. I stretched and breathed, breathed and stretched, until my body was able to let go of tightness and tension.

Although I was mostly focused on bodily sensation during this time, I started to experience a slowing down of the mind as well. I felt mentally calmer—like I was good enough, like I was going home.

This was the beginning of two tectonic shifts in the way I approached training. The first was the idea that if I was listening to my body, I could better adjust my practice. The second idea was that a relaxed body together with a calm mind was much more effective for making progress. I was learning to move with the cycles.

My new discovery began to influence not only my method of training, but also my way of being. My routine was like this: after nine hours of sleep, I'd wake up and have a light breakfast. Then I'd mobilize, shower, have lunch, take a nap. Once rested, I'd make the drive to De Anza Jr College in Cupertino, where I had free access (a necessity in the pauper existence of an amateur athlete) to the throwing ring and weight room.

The discus world-record holder John Powell had a condo about five minutes from campus, so often before my workout I'd head over to his place. There I'd hang out with a bunch of bright, easygoing track and field athletes and, with a sixteen-ounce glass of that awful instant iced tea in hand, I'd do another thirty minutes of body mobilization before heading to the college to start my day of work: throwing the shot.

My workout was comprised of forty to seventy throws, varying each day depending on my energy and whether I was able to get into the groove. Some days I had lots of energy while other days I had little. My training with Ralph had taught me that the mind can override the body; this was useful at that time, but in San Jose I decided to temper that lesson. As my mind and body were becoming less rigid and more open, I began to truly pay attention. On one of those low-energy days, or when I was just feeling crappy, after a lousy round of throws I would take a twenty minute break to reset, then start again. All the while I was doing my new practice of observing and adapting.

My new relaxed mental and physical state quickly began to pay off. The previous stagnation lifted and I was throwing farther with less tension and mental strife. And, more importantly, it was beginning to be fun again. With about a year to go until the Olympic Trials, things were looking up and I could see around the bend in the road—it lay out before me open and clear.

YOU GOT TO WANT TO KNOW

Spiritual teacher Ken Russell (I'll talk more about him later) had a recurring question he'd ask when trying to determine my internal state. He'd say, "So…what's going on?"

Pretty simple, but pretty poignant. What *is* going on?

Being curious about what's happening—how you feel, what your body needs—is the starting point. Often times, this curiosity happens only after things go wrong. When life's going swimmingly, why ask why? But when things aren't so great—you throw out your back, you get a less-than-ideal score on your cholesterol test, you can no longer button your pants—that's usually when people start to want to know what's happening. For me, initially it was when I just couldn't seem to make progress in my throws. Adversity helps promote curiosity. So, whatever is motivating you to make changes in your life, being curious is the best place to start.

WHAT'S GOING ON WITH YOU?

Your body is always saying something. So be curious—it's up to you to find out what that is.

When I'm working with a client, I always start a session by asking a few questions. When I'm not around to check in, I encourage folks to question themselves. Of course, every now and then I make the mistake of asking "How do you feel?" Bad coach. Why? Because most say, "Fine"—even when that's not really the case.

General statements and vague answers just aren't that helpful. To get more specific, here are a few of my favorites:

> *How does my body feel?*
> *How's my energy?*
> *How do my joints feel?*
> *How much sleep did I get last night?*
> *What's my stress level?*
> *Am I hungry?*
> *What's my mood?*

Go ahead and ask. This is the beginning of knowing yourself.

LISTEN UP! HEAR SOMETHING?

Now that you've asked, it's time to pay attention to the answer. And I mean the real answer: not the one you think you're supposed to have or the one you'd like to have or the one you had yesterday.

Here's where I plug meditation. There are a million reasons to meditate. These include, but are not limited to: getting better at focusing, learning how to pay attention, and having the opportunity to listen in a less distracted way. This is not some woo-woo ethereal practice;

meditation is a wholly practical way to train the mind. Through the practice of meditation (or sitting quietly, taking a moment, pausing—whatever you want to call it) you'll be able to better pay attention to the voice of your body, and you might be able to do so while simultaneously filtering all your old beliefs and judgments about what it's telling you.

So take a moment. Sit back, relax, and listen.

JUDGE NOT/YOU ARE NOT A WEENIE

Now that you're listening, you may discover that you don't always like what you hear. Taking a nonjudgmental approach is critical to making change. Of course, you could spend a lot of time and energy avoiding and/or beating yourself up about what your body is telling you, but that's time and energy that could definitely be better spent.

So, you've paused for a moment to listen to your body. Lots of things might come up—sensations, thoughts, emotions. This is where you take a step back and do your best (and goodness knows it ain't easy!) to look at what's happening with a bit of neutrality.

During this stage, it's good to remind yourself of this: You are not a weenie.

This is important because we (specifically, our egos) tend to want to push through, push against, power over. This was a big problem for me—for years, I thought that I had to "man up," meaning I needed to ignore my body and its needs for the sake of always pushing harder, working harder, straining harder. But when I started to let go of my desire to control each and every damn thing each and every damn day, I was able to approach my body with less judgment and approach my life with more patience and intelligence. And I accomplished more and felt better, too.

Often when I plan a workout with clients, they'll say something like, "Oh, I'm OK. My body aches, my joints hurt, I've got a slight cold, I haven't slept well the last few days, and I just broke up with my fiancée. But let's just push through it." Does this work? Answer: Nope. If that's your approach, then you're not really paying attention. And if you're getting caught up in that whole "shut up and buck up" attitude, you might want to ask yourself: What, exactly, is the point? Does everybody have to think you're tough all the time? And, finally: How's that working for you?

IT IS WHAT IT IS.

So the universe has a plan for you that's different than *your* plan for you? Yeah, them's the breaks. You could spend a lot of time fighting it, but ultimately that's like hitting your head against a concrete wall— it's not going to change anything and it's going to give you a hell of a headache.

Once you've truly listened to your body—while tracking your judgments and trying not to become attached to them—then you have options for what to do. I think going with the flow is the best choice, because ultimately that's the only choice that's going to give you peace of mind. Practicing acceptance may not be easy, but it is far and away the most cost efficient—less pain and suffering, less striving and struggling; more ease and calm, more feelings of success.

As my friend Dennis Kelly likes to say, "It is what it is—and it's all good."

THE EXPERIMENT—FINDING WHAT WORKS FOR YOU

Here's where you try things out. Your body, your life, your self is the perfect lab. You get to experiment to figure out what works best—day to day and year to year.

Here's one method: Start your workout. You begin running, kickboxing, yoga, whatever. The first five minutes, plan to be totally open. Use those five minutes to follow steps one through four of the energy output scale from the previous chapter (p. 24). Maybe you discover that your energy is low and that you need to back off. Or you might find that you've got an extra kick and you could pick it up a notch. Using whatever information you've gathered, determine if what you'd been planning for your workout is going to be the kindest and most productive choice, or if you need to modify. Either you can stick with the plan or make a new one. Regardless—it's all good.

REPEAT

I won't mention that cliché about change, but I will say this: everything's changing. All the time. The only constant thing, etc. This ain't a one-time deal; you've got to stick with it for, well, ever, and therefore moving through these four steps is a lifetime gig. Repeat!

BRUTALLY HONEST MEANS DON'T BS YOURSELF

A few years ago I worked with Jamie Moyer, a Major League Baseball pitcher with a successful twenty-five-year career. In 2012, he pitched and won a game at the age of forty-nine. In doing so he set an MLB record as the oldest player to win a game. One day recently, talking over coffee and donuts at Top Pot Doughnuts in Seattle, he was in a reflective mood. He told me that one of the things he had learned in our time together was that he needed to be "brutally honest" with himself. He's always been known as a fierce competitor with a strong work ethic, and he took pride in out-working his fellow baseball players. He had been of the mindset to just buck up and push through despite fatigue or injury, but during his last few years playing ball, he began to check in more (with a little nudging from me). Jamie realized that his strategy wasn't working for him like it had in his early years, and so he adapted, changing his game plan to not only bolster his day-to-day performance but also to set him up for longevity, for sustaining his fitness for the rest of life.

Not just successful elite athletes will benefit from this approach. In our modern-day frazzled and fast-paced culture, many hold the belief that to push hard, work hard, strive hard all the time is necessary to achieve success. In fact, the belief is so strong that many choose to just opt out because they believe that if they can't do everything then why bother doing anything. We are primed for the sixty-hour work week starting in childhood—I've trained with teenagers who have highly structured schedules, jam packed with school, homework, sports, and extra-curricular activities. The competition has become cutthroat, and the idea that more equals better is causing young people a great deal of stress. These kids are learning early on to not listen to their bodies, to not pay attention to their energy, and to allow external standards and expectations to guide their lives. The end result: exhausted, burnt-out teens becoming exhausted burnt-out adults.

Many of us are starting to suspect that our diseases and conflicts are, if not 100 percent proven to be caused by stress, then at a minimum highly correlated with it. As an Olympic competitor working to reach excellence, I had to learn that the model of push more, work more, strive more was not only counter-productive in terms of my athletic goals but also in terms of my health. As a coach, I've come to encourage my clients to evaluate the exercise programs at their health clubs and gyms that push people to their limits all the time, every time. I'm sure the thinking is that you will make greater gains more quickly by pushing yourself every single day, by being relentless, and by ignoring yourself when your mind or body is calling *uncle*. But I've found that this mentality hurts more than it helps, and I've learned from first-hand experience that it simply does not work. Going with the cycles of the body yields greater results.

My advice, therefore, is to be cautious about those who sell quick fixes and fast results gained through constantly pushing beyond your current cycle of energy. Instead, pay attention to your ever-changing energy levels, moods, and mental vacillations, and let that information guide you. Only you can determine the best course to feel more vital, be happier, and enjoy a more balanced life.

If you know the enemy and know yourself,
you need not fear the result of a hundred battles.
SUN TZU, THE ART OF WAR

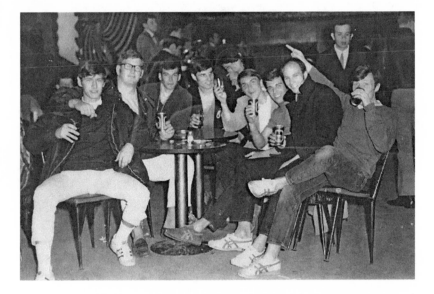

Juarez Mexico, 1970. Spring break party time with Oregon teammates.
(I'm second from the left; the iconic runner Steve Prefontaine is fourth from the right)

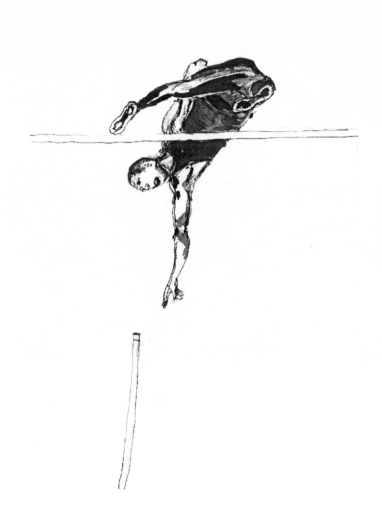

The supreme art of war is to subdue the enemy without fighting.

SUN TZU, THE ART OF WAR

A CALM MIND IS A MOBILE MIND

Let's pretend for a moment that we're football players. You happen to be the running back, like Seattle's beloved Marshawn Lynch. You're on the field, crouched in your stance, ready to go into beast mode. The quarterback hands you the ball…now, if you want to do your job, you'd better be sure that your eyes are wide open and focused, because there's a bunch of professional athletes charging you, big burly guys who want nothing more than to take you out. If you're not aware of what's coming, you'll end up on the ground, breathless and crushed flat. Your success—in this case, your ability to avoid harm—depends on having a clear picture of what's coming so that you can utilize all the skills you've spent years practicing. You're present, you're focused, and you're strong. If you can do and be all that, then you'll be headed toward a touchdown.

Having a mobile mind is about being able to observe and create space around the ongoing, never-ending bombardment of thoughts. Like a running back having a wide-angle view of the defense, it's essential to see one's thoughts as clearly as possible, and from that position make smart, productive choices. Obviously, this metaphor is a bit on the simplistic side—your thoughts are neither on the opposing or the home team. They simply exist, and it's up to you to figure out which is which. And, after a lot of years of habitual thinking, trying to make this discernment can be like being in a bad marriage: sometimes it's hard to tell what's love and what's somebody tearing you down.

At a certain point in my life, my relationship with my thinking had gotten so bad that I was about ready for a divorce. But with the luck of having some really great teachers and some unique experiences, I was able to learn a little mental nonviolent communication and find a way to better deal with it. I developed what I began to call a "mobile mind": having both mental flexibility and strength, plus the ability to see the pothole in the road and avoid it. It's keeping quiet and calm within pandemonium, control within chaos. It's about not fighting but not giving in, like a palm tree bending in the wind without breaking.

Since everyone has a mind, you know that its messages are about 80 percent nonsense and 10 percent bullshit. Thoughts are not necessarily reality, no matter how many times you think them—if you take your thoughts personally, they're in control; if you don't, they aren't. Mobile mind is the work of cultivating mental strength, working toward a better understanding of your thinking patterns, and learning to use your mind wisely. Knowing the mental landscape is essential, and working to exert a little healthy control will give you that peace of mind. And it'll make your life easier, too.

BATTLING MYSELF AND MOBILIZING MY MIND

Pervasive negative thoughts began entering my mind during my freshman year of college, gaining momentum each passing year. By the time I was training in San Jose at the age of twenty-four, if I didn't get it right (no matter what it was), my internal monologue would default to horrible self-talk, like a dictator reprimanding a lowly subject. It didn't matter what I did, how well I did it, or if there was any improvement. If what I was doing wasn't done *perfectly*, I would berate myself till the cows came home. I had absolutely no mercy on myself.

"What the fuck?" I'd yell. "Why can't you do this? Just do it right and do it now!"

Although I'm sure there were a lot of influences, I think this kind of self-talk had a lot to do with my upbringing. I grew up with an alcoholic mother and an estranged father, and I don't remember my parents ever telling me that I was capable of good things, or great things—or anything really, for that matter. Like most kids do, I internalized my early formative experiences with my caregivers, and over time those external messages morphed into deep feelings of ineptitude and unworthiness, following me into adulthood and taking over my own voice.

So, it was about nine months until the Olympic Trials in July of 1976. With the biggest challenge of my young life getting closer every day, this old bad habit was taking on greater force, and as my excitement over the possibility of making the Olympic team amped up, so too did the power of my self-destructive thoughts.

Basically, instead of getting pumped about this extraordinary opportunity, I was freaking out. My anxious thinking was sucking the joy out of everything, dousing any sense of accomplishment and killing my hope. It's like suddenly I had partial amnesia, forgetting everything I had learned before with Ralph, Bill, and Al—forgetting previous successes and recalling only past failures, and I didn't seem to be able to escape the vice-like grip my destructive thoughts had on me.

Physically, I am a pretty quick and sure-footed guy. But at this time, mentally I was a mess, getting stuck in repetitive chatter about my general unworthiness and the certainty of my failure. I'd have these waves of chaotic, derogatory, angry thoughts; at times, these destructive mental surges would arrive in tidal wave proportion. I had the choice to flow with the wave, paddle faster, catch up to it and ride, baby, ride—or be held under the surface and get crushed by the wave's massive force.

I needed help, and I needed help fast. Funny thing was, my physical training was evolving nicely. I was getting faster and stronger every day, but meanwhile my mind was being a real pain in the ass. Even though a part of me knew that those negative thoughts weren't really true, a bigger part of me was still listening to them. Then a third part of me was hating myself for listening, and a fourth part of me was identifying with them. Lots of wasted energy there. So despite making progress in some ways, I was unable to find the eye of that mental storm, instead getting whipped around like a rag doll in a hurricane.

I needed something to grab on to—a signpost, a map, a solid piece of advice. Lucky for me, books have always had a way of finding me in my hour of need. The first time this happened was when I was a teenager and stumbled on *Psycho-Cybernetics*, by Maxwell Maltz, which pointed to the human mind's ability to generate thoughts that can take us down to the lowest lows, but also the mind's potential to lift us up, shift perspectives, and create change. I absorbed the message at the time, just clearly not enough, and at twenty-four, I still struggled. Just when it seemed that I'd be stuck forever in a torturous mental prison, W. Timothy Gallwey's *The Inner Game of Tennis* found me in the nick of time.

A favorite quote of mine is, "To be aware is to be awake." Up to this point in my athletic career, I had been asleep in many ways, ways that could keep me from my dream of making the Olympic team. *The Inner Game of Tennis* was a giant wake-up call, an alarm clock for my drowsy psyche.

From the very first page, it was like I couldn't read fast enough. Gallwey wrote about two competing selves: first, the maniacal, self-berating one, which likes to maintain an ongoing dialogue of self-blame and criticism; and a second, kinder, more accepting one, which is better able to observe what's happening with compassion and forgiveness. It was easy for me to recognize my most dominate self, and unfortunately that one was one grumpy bastard. The nice one was notably absent.

Gallwey, it seemed, was talking straight to me. I read his book every day, and soon I realized how distant I'd become from my compassionate and forgiving self. His words, like arrows, hit a direct shot into the heart of the matter, pinpointing exactly how I treated myself. My self-deprecating mantra wasn't working any longer, and finding this book helped me to see my patterns of destructive self-talk, putting me back on a more positive emotional track and granting me permission to accept myself as I was. This lesson, although not totally new but apparently forgotten, was an important and profound lesson—and very difficult to fully integrate. Old habits die hard, and, like I've mentioned before, I have a long habit of "more is more" and "push till you drop" that all my practices had yet to permanently unseat. Reading this book was a moment of solace, a sigh of relief, a letting myself off the hook—I felt that someone understood my experience and sympathized, and that gave me some peace.

I had really taken Gallwey's message to heart, and soon I integrated it into my training sessions, too. I'd already started to become more emotionally balanced in general, and now I didn't get overly excited by a successful weightlifting session, or become downtrodden by a throw coming up short. Instead of reacting to a less-than-optimal performance with anger and shame, I began to observe things from a different perspective that, slowly and with practice, became less judgmental. Of course the thoughts still came. After an imperfect throw, I'd catch myself thinking, *That was some shitty throw* or *Why can't you just do it right?* In the past, I would've poured fuel on the fire, getting madder and madder, fanning my mental anguish. But because of the book, I started to be more agile in flicking those thoughts off me like an ember from a campfire—I didn't allow my thoughts and self-criticism to stay and burn. And since I gave them less power by not paying attention to them, they started to have less of an effect on me.

Sometimes I'd simply stop my training session and breathe. During these "timeouts" I'd try to analyze what'd just taken place, then come up with a new game plan. This method would help me for the next twenty-five years, and it'd be reinforced when, decades later, I met Ken Russell, my awareness and meditation teacher.

I got to put this all into practice at De Anza College, my new training home. I had distanced myself from the other shot putters at San Jose State College, as well as the action-packed downtown San Jose YMCA, because I wanted to be less distracted by the banter and constant "who's doing what" gossip of the San Jose group. A couple of guys—Brian Oldfield, the first shot putter to sign up for the short-lived professional track circuit, and John Powell, the American record holder in the discus at the time—co-anchored the De Anza throwing crew with me. They, too, wanted to get away from the mayhem of the larger group.

Brian was one of the greatest athletes I've ever known. He was big—6'5" and 275 lb.—and could move like a cat, simultaneously graceful and explosive. His presence was bigger than life in the most positive sense; he was just one of those people who could suck you into his force field, then motivate you to push yourself beyond your limits. John, on the other hand, was quiet and more internally focused. Besides being a record holder he was also a cop; in his uniform he was an imposing figure, and on the field he wore a protective shell that worked to keep people—and the distractions they bring—at bay. Despite John's seeming aloofness, he was a great practice partner, extending himself to suggest that every time I had the insidious thought "I can't," I must repeat ten times "I can." This advice (the phrasing of which I later expanded to "I can do it"), and the lessons that unfolded within this positive environment (along with the fact that I wasn't competing against either of these guys), helped me to make the great strides needed to get me to the Olympics.

With these guys on my side, the ten-mile drive from San Jose to De Anza College in Cupertino began to take on an enjoyable anticipation. Thoughts of *Wow, this is going to be a great day!* flooded my mind on the drive. Brian and John had such skill in positive thinking that, by working alongside them, my own thinking was becoming calmer and much less critical—my mind was becoming more mobile. These two guys, both senior to me by a few years, were encouraging me to go beyond my physical limits while maintaining my mellow, and because of them my performance was actually improving. Plus, every day before practice I would read the first chapter of *The Inner Game of Tennis* and then implement its message into my throws. With Gallwey's directive freshly imprinted in mind, I'd head out to the practice field feeling less internal pressure than before and with the sense that I could better control my mind. This new mental agility gave me strength, strength that allowed me to dodge the harmful thoughts that had been plaguing me and holding me back.

One day, Brian and I were throwing together when he called it quits. Instead of heading out, he decided to stand outside the landing area and cheer me on. I was throwing a light shot of 14 lb. (instead of the regular 16 lb.), in order to work on speed. At that weight, my best throw had been about 72' thus far, but in that moment, with Brian cheering me on, it felt like no one existed but us two, and I was able to harness a new calm but powerful force.

Throw by throw I improved—first a 73' throw, then a couple of 74' throws. Brian stood a foot beyond my last throw, yelling, "Hit me, Peter! Hit me!" And each time I released the shot put, I'd somehow throw farther in my attempt to reach him. He was now standing 76' from me, and before I let go of the shot, I silently whispered within my mind, *I can do it.* As I released the final throw, it felt as though the shot put was flying effortlessly, supercharged by a mind that was as strong as it was calm.

Thankfully I didn't actually hit Brian, but I did reach the 76' mark where he stood. Wide-eyed, he leapt in celebration of my throw.

A few weeks later, I headed north to my hometown of Eugene, Oregon for one of the last big meets before the Olympic Trials. The meet was the Prefontaine Classic, named after Steve Prefontaine, a legend-to-be and one of the greatest long distance runners of his era. In the Prefontaine Classic, I was competing in front of a friendly home crowd, knowledgeable spectators who supported all former University of Oregon graduates with enthusiastic applause.

Rather than doing my old jumping-around-and-yelling method of getting psyched that usually put me in an adrenaline-fueled frenzy, I did the practice I'd put together over the past two years—doing my self-created stretching exercises and a breathing meditation alone and in the quietest place possible. Before the Prefontaine, I took fifteen minutes to set my body and mind right through a calm, deliberate practice. Soon enough it was time to head out to the field to warm up and, with my name ringing over the loudspeaker, join the competition.

A half hour and six throws later, I had a new personal record of 69'3". But the best part was that it was the easiest throw of my life.

IT. WAS. THE. EASIEST. THROW. OF. MY. LIFE.

I did not achieve this success through harsh, punitive directives or destructive self-talk—I'd done it because of years of physical training combined with a new mental focus and a belief that resounded in every cell of my body that *I can do it.*

From this moment on, my life changed. Not just because I'd thrown my best throw, but because I saw how powerful a calm and mobile mind can truly be. I began applying this reality in all areas of my life. And it made all the difference.

HOW TO MAKE YOUR MIND MOBILE

Take a Break

Put down the phone, turn off the TV, take off the headphones. When difficult thoughts arise, don't run away and don't get distracted. An infinity of apps will not save you. Again, a plug here for meditation. Be still, be quiet. See what happens.

Recognize

If you don't see negative thinking, then you can't change it. The first key to mental mobility is to recognize your problematic thinking as such. If you're standing on the field with your eyes shut tight, you're not going to be able to see the defensive end heading toward you. But when you pay attention to what's happening, you can better see what's coming.

We all have thoughts that attempt to get the best of us. In many cases, these thoughts are old ones we have yet to shed, even though they are not serving us. Old, negative internal narratives reside quietly but potently in the subconscious, only to randomly awaken at inopportune

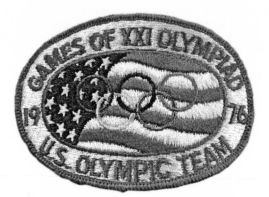

moments and cause us to question our self-worth. Recognizing that phenomenon is the first—and most important—step to managing it.

Get to Know Your Mind

Another football analogy: Now that you've decided to get in the game, you can prepare yourself. The only way to do that is to study the other team, to figure out how they play so that you'll know how to respond. And even if the opposing team's coach holds the clipboard up in front of his face so that you can't get direct information about what's coming next, over time and with patience you'll begin to understand the patterns of plays.

Study your dark thoughts so that you can work with them. To do this, write them down. Label them. Hell, name them. ("Oh, looks like Angry Dad is here today.") The point is to learn about them so that when they come at you, you know what move to make to avoid being blindsided.

Don't Go There

When negative self-talk rears its ugly head, apply the "don't go there" technique. Although there's no way to stop a thought, you can decide not to follow it. There are lots of schools of thought on this matter, two of which are in the forefront of current American study and practice. The first is a wonderful method often associated with cognitive behavioral therapy. This is what John Powell's method of "I can" was tapping into—every time you notice an unkind thought emerging, first recognize it, then replace it with something else. You aren't trying to push a thought away or pretend like it's not there; you're simply teaching your mind to do something different, something more likely to make you feel good and help you do good in the world.

Use my "I can do it " mantra, or pick something else. It can be affirming or neutral—what it is matters less than the fact that you are choosing not to indulge those tired old thoughts. Because life's hard enough without your own mind bumming you out.

Watch It

The second method, often associated with the practice of mindfulness, takes a less active but just as effective approach. It goes something like this: the thought, do nothing, repeat. Remember how I used to fuel that self-shaming fire by ranting and raving every time I didn't make a perfect throw? That's the opposite of this. Instead of scolding yourself, just...don't. And when the inevitable happens—when you scold yourself, then scold yourself for scolding yourself, and on and on like the reflection in a roomful of mirrors—instead of scolding yourself for scolding yourself, just watch it happen. Thoughts do their thing, prompted or randomly. Just watch them. Notice the thoughts, and notice the emotions that can come up with them. Then let both the thought and the feeling around the thought do their thing and fade away.

Practice

That's it—just practice.

Seek a Calm and Strong Mind

Your mind is a wonderful tool, and the more you study it the better you can use it. A calm mind is a strong mind, and a strong mind has the power to create a more peaceful, more effective life.

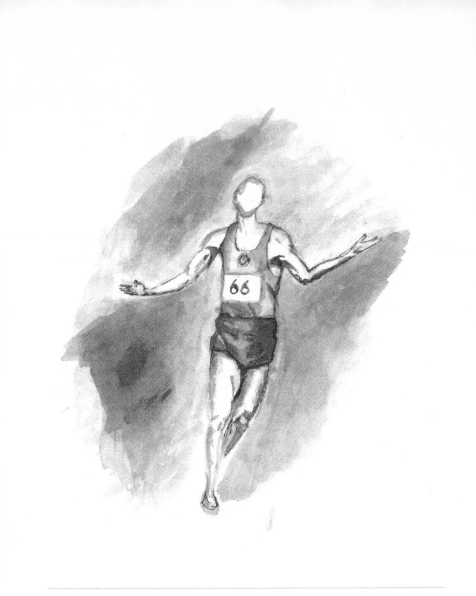

There is one way of breathing that is shameful and constricted. Then, there's another way: a breath of love that takes you all the way to infinity.

RUMI

ALLOWING

There you are, poised with your bow and arrow. Today, it seems, you're into archery. Your feet are planted shoulder-width apart, solid and strong on the ground, and the muscles of your legs are firm but relaxed, ready for anything. Your left arm is straight, your left hand gripping the bow, and your right hand holds the arrow true against the breeze. As you pull the arrow back, the bowstring taut, you look down the line of the arrow toward the target. A bead of sweat rolls across your hairline and down your forehead, the anticipation building with the tension of the string. And then you release the arrow, and there's nothing left to do but let go.

In that moment, as the arrow begins its trajectory through space, you've relinquished all control over the situation, all control over the outcome. You've done what's needed to be done, practicing for days, months, years, visualizing and adjusting and returning again and again. You've acted. Now, once the arrow is released, all you can do is wait, and allow to happen whatever is going to happen.

At this point, all the willpower or hope or desire in the universe will not make a difference; you won't know how it will turn out until the arrow hits the target. The only thing to do is to do nothing but wait, be still; anything more is a waste of time and energy.

For a lucky few, this moment after the work's finished is an opportunity to relax. You can shrug your shoulders, say to yourself, "I did my best," and pour yourself a celebratory beer. For many, however, the waiting is an anxiety producer. Either way, what's done is done: whether it works out for you or not, you've pursued your goal as far as you can. What happens next is out of your hands.

I call that in-between moment, that moment after the cause and before the effect, "allowing." If you're anything like me, you like the action part more than the allowing part. But you gotta have both. When I was younger, I felt that the action part was where the real progress was being made, and the non-action part was just a damn huge waste of time. But, alas, after the egg has been laid, you have to wait for it to hatch. That chick isn't going to grow by your pacing, or worrying, or trying to will it into being with your mind. It's going to grow because that's what it does—it grows. Without you. Because you're not the boss of the universe.

The athlete who decides that rest and recovery are as valuable as effort is steps ahead of the rest of the pack. And the athlete who's fine-tuned her skill at "allowing" is one step beyond that—the mysterious process of repair and regeneration usually happens when nothing else is going on.

Friend and *New York Times* best-selling author Garth Stein once told me about his writing practice. After his morning work session, he spends some quiet time away from whatever he's created. This, he claims, allows him to see what he's put on paper in a way he couldn't have done during the actual act of writing. For him, if he struggles to make something happen, to force a word or idea, the very thing he seeks to accomplish eludes him. Instead, he stays in the pause for a while; he simply steps away and allows his writing to rest, like well-kneaded dough resting so that it can rise. Then when he returns, he's in a different mind space and oftentimes he can see something that he wasn't able to see before.

The same thing can happen when we are at the starting point and simply trying to figure out the next step. There are those glorious moments in life when the path forward rings clear as a bell; and there are moments when the path is covered by shadow and you're wearing sunglasses. We've all been in situations where, despite well-planned and neatly orchestrated effort, we're unable to make headway. And there are those hard moments when confusion stops us before we even have a chance to begin. Those are the moments when this age-old adage comes in handy: sometimes the best way out of something is through it.

SOMETIMES YOU JUST HAVE TO STOP

I placed ninth in the 1976 Montreal Olympics, but instead of relishing the moment, about two seconds after I stepped off the field I was itching to compete again, All I really wanted to do was take a couple days off, then go to the next Olympics, without having to do off-season training or participate in all those in-between meets or, really, wait.

The three-and-a-half years following were the worst of my life. I struggled on every level, both personally and in terms of my performance. I'd gotten married right after the Olympics, but two years in my new wife left to pursue her career. I was on my own, sweating every month to make ends meet while trying to manage my increasing discontent and boredom. Plus, I spent all that time working hard—and had almost nothing to show for it. With the 1980 trials looming ahead and my perceived failures following behind, I decided to give myself an ultimatum. Obviously I was still a "more is more" kinda guy at heart. So, for a meet in Berkeley six weeks before the trials, I set a goal for myself: to throw the shot 67'. If I reached that mark, then maybe I could launch myself out of my stagnation and lose the sense of futility that haunted me—maybe even get a little more hopeful about my chances. If I wasn't able to reach that mark, then I'd quit.

It had been a long four years to get to that point in Berkeley in 1980, and my anxiety around my lack of improvement was growing. Over the previous year, I had sought out various coaches and teachers to help me find the reason why I wasn't performing well. I'd traveled to Houston to train with Tom Tellez, an Olympic coach who'd coached Carl Lewis, the 100-meter gold medalist. He had really helped me hone my technique prior to the 1976 Olympic Trials and I thought he could work his magic again. Yet, that too didn't work. I looked everywhere, searching for the technique, the trick that would set things back on track. I was looking for answers. And I was coming up with nothing.

Setting that ultimatum helped to keep me focused—until I stepped into the ring and failed to meet my goal at all six throws. Afterward, I decided that even though the Olympic Trials were only six weeks away, I would not be attending. I was quitting.

After that horrific meet, I went home to my dank and shabby little apartment, a few blocks away from the ocean in Huntington Beach. For the next three days, I stayed in and did nothing. I simply sat on my couch with my pit bull, Buck, by my side. I fed him. I walked him on the beach, watching the waves brush the shore. Other than that, I did nothing. I lay there. I just stopped. I didn't try to make any plans or figure out how to pull myself together. I decided that it was over and I just sat quietly, in silence. I was actually able to find a little peace in the pain, certain that this period of my life had come to an end.

On the third day, an idea entered my head like a lightning bolt. Out of nowhere and completely unexpected—BOOM!—there it was. Remember, I was done searching for an answer, not trying to fix my throwing, not trying to solve anything. I'd surrendered, giving up my need not only to alleviate the situation but to understand, even deciding to simply move on with my life. I'd thought that all those years of hard work, all those almosts, were over.

And then suddenly that big idea flashed into my head. I recognized this thought—it was one I'd had years ago, which at the time I'd discarded like a piece of junk mail. It must've been way back in some dusty crevice of my mind, lying dormant. Apparently, its hibernation period was complete. The barren winter had ended and an unexpected spring had come.

I'll spare you the technical details, but basically the thought was about that technique I'd stopped searching for, a technique for creating the perfect and most efficient throw. It combined the best aspects of Al Feuerbach's and George Wood's throwing techniques, melded into something that I hoped would create a better rhythm that would specifically fit me. It'd been there all along, but I'd been looking, going in another direction. Giving up—staying still—had allowed the answer to find me.

With that idea in mind, I went out to an empty, unfamiliar track. I went there not to throw, but to mull it over, to play with the idea without actually acting on it. I just imagined the technique. It felt good. It felt natural. It had a rhythm to it that I hadn't experienced for years.

I went home. I allowed more thoughts to surface about it, but I didn't actively contemplate it; I just let it simmer.

The next day I returned to the same track. This time, I threw the shot—not far, not half the distance I could have, but with a sense of lightness and play, this new idea, new technique, and new rhythm in mind. The ideas came and I followed their prompting. I rediscovered my groove and recovered the part of myself that'd given up. That said, I still had no thoughts of throwing my hat back into the Olympic Trials ring.

Every day following this moment of inspiration, I gained a bit more confidence. My throws started to feel easier and more natural. My panic was gone; there was a sense of relaxation, of letting go of agenda and trusting stillness. So I decided to implement a game plan to move forward, with the possibility of the Olympic Trials back on the table. But unlike my former strict ultimatums, this plan stemmed from a deeper resolve, a belief in myself and my ability to see my hard work through.

THE DRY SPELL ENDS

A couple of weeks later there was a national championship meet at UCLA, and I decided that this would be the time to throw my hat back into the ring. I flew down to UCLA, ready with my new technique and a calm determination. I placed third out of twelve, with my best finish and best throw of the last four years. It felt good. Really good. Even though a few weeks earlier I'd been sure I had no chance, now going to the Olympic Trials seemed like the right thing to do. I let everyone know that I was back and that I would meet them in Eugene in just a few weeks.

On the outside, I was able to maintain my cool and calm demeanor. But as I flew into Eugene, my internal landscape was starting to buckle under the pressure. The voices of my old companions— those catastrophic thoughts—echoed in my head, getting louder and ruder by the minute. *Where the hell did these guys come from?* I wondered.

Once I arrived on campus, I headed to the dormitories that would soon house all of us athletes. Lucky for me, these were the same dorms that I had lived in ten years earlier, so I was familiar with the environment and therefore had one less thing to worry about. I still knew my way around, and it still felt like home.

I acquired the Olympic Trials event program, reading the articles analyzing the participants and their upcoming events. Under my event the various throwers were listed with their pre-ranking and odds of making the team. At the bottom of the list, next to my name, were the words: *May be past his prime.*

"Fuck you," I said, then quickly remembered not to go negative. Redirecting, I murmured, "Quiet. Don't go there."

While I didn't want the tension that the anger reaction could create in my body, for a moment the anger felt good, like encountering an old friend. But I knew the effect would not serve me if I stayed in it too long, so I guided my thinking to focus on the events ahead.

After the roller coaster ride of the past few weeks, I had no expectation about making it onto the top-three podium, which would be necessary to make the Olympic Team. I had no thought of winning, and no real thought of losing either.

That experience of desperation, allowing, and inspiration changed the course of my career and, of course, my life. It changed the course of everything. I'd once believed wholeheartedly that I was driving, I was making it happen, that I was in charge. On that lonely third day in my beachside apartment, with only Buck and my despair keeping me company, I received a gift that allowed me to question all my fundamental beliefs about how to find the way when I'm lost. It truly rocked my inflated ego, my naïve belief that I had all the answers—or that I had any answers at all, for that matter. To this day, I know that I was not responsible for the change; rather, I had unintentionally placed myself in a space of surrender, and from that, allowed something to come forward. It was a gift, a surprising and graceful one. But where did it come from? Beats me. If I had to name it, I'd call it the "Great Whatever." Because it's not something, it's nothing. And how am I supposed to name nothing?

ACTION + ALLOWING

Here we bump up against a paradox. How do you allow? You stop striving, stop trying to control, stop deluding yourself that your effort directly affects your gains. The fact that my failure and subsequent loss of hope led to inspiration and accomplishment is not the point. Sometimes that happens; often it doesn't. But I do believe in "having a gut feeling," in the possibility of accessing an internal sense of how to move forward in life. You just can't think you're way through everything all of the time. Even Spock couldn't come up with a solution every time (he was half human, after all). If, like most of us, you succumb to ideologies, expectations, and norms created by the culture-at-large, it's likely that sometimes external influences override your own ability to deal with your situation. Since thoughts are usually echoes of something someone told you, using your mind to reason your way to a different, creative answer just won't always work.

In short, allowing requires stopping, sitting, and doing nothing, with NO agenda that such stopping, sitting, and doing nothing is going to get you anywhere. If you stop and sit because you think that's going to get results, then you are doing the exact same thing you were doing before, just in a different color.

ADMIT TO I DON'T KNOW

Maybe you tried something and it didn't work out. Maybe you tried everything and that didn't work out either. This is that hard moment, when you have to admit something terrible: YOU DON'T KNOW. You do not have the answer. If you did, you'd have figured it out by now. In that moment, you may feel like you're caught in a vortex of confusion; you may feel disappointed and uncomfortably humbled. And that's OK.

BE OK WITH NOT KNOWING

Now, let go of your agenda, including your agenda not to have an agenda. For us type-A folks, the admission of not knowing is damn hard, but being OK with it can be damn harder. But since it's happening anyway, you might as well be OK with it, right?

TAKE A BREAK FROM ASKING OTHERS FOR THE ANSWER

You've spent a lot of time asking other people for an answer. You asked your coach, your best friend, your grandma, the teenager who bags your groceries. You've read every blog, newsletter, and magazine you can possibly think of. You've bought in bulk from the bookstore's self-help section, and you've paid through the nose for expert advice from people who claim to have the answer.

But it's now clear that "they" don't have the answer. So stop asking them.

TAKE A BREAK FROM ASKING YOURSELF (AKA YOUR MIND) FOR THE ANSWER

This one is tricky. It's that whole "don't think about a pink elephant" thing. For me, pre-1980 Olympic Trials, I'd basically reached such a level of despair that I'd come to terms with not knowing. I'd given up on an answer entirely. So that's kinda what you have to do: give up. Or, for a more positive reframe: take a break. Just like after an intense work you need to rest your body in order to recover, your brain needs a rest too. The question has been asked, and you've worked hard to find an answer. Now, chill out. If you can get out of the way for a second, you might be surprised by what emerges.

TAKE A BREAK FROM DISTRACTIONS

So you've decided to stop asking. It'd be easy to immediately fill that empty space in your day with distractions, but just don't do it. I'm talking any number of things: booze, social media, sex, sugar, TV. Books, bars, drugs, company. Filling up your calendar. Cranking up the music. Working too much. Playing too hard. Surfing the internet. Whatever your distraction go-to is, take a break from it, too. Let there be room in your life for something new to arrive.

BE...QUIET

During those three days, I'd stopped asking. I'd given up. I had surrendered. For the first time in my life I wasn't in control and there was nothing left to do but sit on my couch next to my dog (I'd stopped asking him, too) and be. Basically, I'd stripped my life of all the things that had been taking me away from—rather than closer to—the answers. What started as nothing became the faintest of whispers, and because of that calm quiet I was able to hear it.

So get quiet.

TRUST

Sit tight. Now is the time to listen, and trust that your inner coach will come through. You won't know what the message is going to be, but rest assured that something's gotta give. This takes a little big-picture thinking, some meditation on the strange and inexplicable experience of being alive. Hey, the world works in mysterious ways.

How can I—or anyone else—tell you how to "allow"? For me, I got to that place because I'd worked really hard and then, despite everything, suffered a great disappointment. I was staring into the abyss, and I let myself fall. And a very lucky thing happened—it turned out OK in the end. That was one moment on my journey; yours will likely be different. You may reach the point where you feel like giving up, and maybe you'll find the answer after surrendering to that. Or you might not get the answer you were counting on or hoping for. Sometimes what comes will feel less like the right path and more like a detour, something unexpected or confusing, even unwelcome. That's OK too. You might not understand it or appreciate it at the time, but that's because the story's not over.

All this to say: there are many really amazing teachers who have lots to offer, and with careful listening and thoughtfulness, you can benefit from their teachings. But no one has the answer, and grasping onto a guru is a fool's errand. So too is scouring your inner landscape for an answer—that's the same search, just turned inward. When it comes down to it, there are many ways to take that next big step, answer your most elusive question, and put a smile on your face. Somewhere inside of you is probably a compass, and whether it's rusty from disuse or perfectly attuned from practice, it will—eventually—show you the way. Ultimately, there's one primary thing you control: when to hang on for dear life, and when to let go. And you never know what might happen or where that free fall might take you.

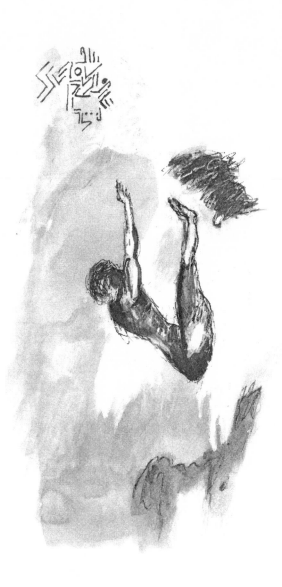

To hold you must first open your hand. Let go.

TAO TE CHING

THE POWER OF CALM

You've probably heard that old British quote: "Keep Calm and Carry On." Threatened by massive German air raids in 1939, England's government was hoping that posters using this phrase would inspire tranquility in the face of everything going to hell. Now, when I think of that phrase—or see it around town in various mutated versions on T-shirts, tote bags, coffee mugs, you name it—it makes me laugh, and reminds me of my high school football days as an offensive lineman.

If football is a metaphor for war (as over the years many have claimed), then my team's pregame ritual certainly didn't follow Her Majesty's advice. It looked something like this: The team would huddle together. Then, we'd jump up and down. Next, we'd yell things like "Yeah, we're gonna get 'em!" and "We're number one!" and "Let's kick these guys' asses!" Then we'd jump up and down some more. The result of this ceremony: we'd get worked up into an adrenaline-fueled, aggression-provoking, unfocused frenzy. We called this "getting psyched up." And it did have that effect. But it also had other effects; usually I'd be somewhat tuckered out from this intense team-bonding moment, and I'd be far from calm. I didn't realize this until years later—all I knew then was that I was drained after our team warm-up and needed time to recover before the start of the game.

Now, if you've ever watched a Quentin Tarantino movie, you know that the first one to lose his cool is the first one to die. If that applied to me and my fellow footballers, we all would've been goners. Fortunately, we weren't facing a vengeful bride with a giant sword. But I did notice that, after the big psyche up, something was "off." Did I eat too much steak before the game? Am I out of shape? Are my shoes tied too tight?

The more frenetic and adrenalized I became before a game, the more I went "up into my head," my mind buzzing with unrelenting thoughts—most of which, true to form, were doubting and anxious and critical. When in my head, I couldn't feel my feet on the ground, and my effectiveness on the field suffered.

A bit later on, I realized that this pre-game energizing was pretty counter-productive. As you may recall from previous chapters, when I reached an elite level of competition, I gave up this ritual and instead focused on creating stillness and quiet in order to prepare for a meet. I knew that getting more hyped-up was the opposite of what I needed to excel. Another step away from indoctrination—I'd discovered that what had been true was no longer (or never had been) true. With that new method of stillness, I had much better results. Calmness was the key—the less my mind interfered the better.

A MYSTICAL ENCOUNTER

Let's return to where I left off in chapter 5, just a few days away from the 1980 Olympic Trials. Although I'd found a new technique out of the depths of despair in which I felt wholly confident, I still had some lingering doubts. I was prepared, but my mind was doing its thing, and I was nervous. Between making the trip to Eugene and discovering my less-than-promising rankings, I'd returned to a riled up state. Trying to soothe my nervousness, I began pacing around campus, swinging back and forth between calm and anxiety, anxiety and calm. Finally, I decided to take a swim, hoping to relieve the tension in my body and mind, and so I headed over to the U of O swimming complex.

It was summer break, so the pool was empty, but I saw someone sitting in the coach's office. I approached and said, "Excuse me, I am wondering if I can use the pool. I'm here to compete in the Olympic Trials."

"Sure, go right ahead," the coach (whose name I've unfortunately forgotten) replied.

So I dove in and swam around a bit. I didn't swim laps; instead, I just kind of moved my body in the water, swirling my legs back and forth in the hopes of loosening up my tense muscles. I was in there for a half hour or so, and I was starting to feel more relaxed in my body. But my mind didn't seem to want to calm down, like a colicky baby who won't stop crying no matter how much you rock him. Feeling like

I'd done all I could do, I got out of the pool and went to say good-bye to the coach.

I'd planned to simply say thank you and head out, but he must've been curious about the big guy floating around in his pool, and he probably sensed my anxiety. Instead of having a quick exchange, he asked me about my practice, and soon we were chatting. The coach was sympathetic to my situation, and told me that he'd long been a student of relaxation and breathing techniques, and that he utilized these techniques in his coaching. He found that it really helped his athletes' performance.

Little did I know then that this would be a moment of learning that would affect me for the rest of my life. Right on time, a teacher had arrived just when I needed one. He kindly offered to teach me his breathing technique, and we agreed to meet the next day.

The next morning at the pool, we set to work. The coach instructed me to lie down somewhere quiet, take a series of normal, regular breaths, and then about every minute or so, take a really deep breath, focusing on a long exhalation. I then repeated that sequence twice more, each time deepening the breath and extending the length of time for both the inhalation and exhalation. At the end, I returned to my normal breathing and just lay there, now in a much better and fuller state of relaxation.

I continued to practice this breathing technique twice daily up to the day of my event. These simple exercises helped me to create distance from my thoughts about the upcoming competition, about whether I was ready, or good enough. My mind became quieter. My new breath training allowed me to get out of my own way once the moment of truth came; it left space in my head, and it allowed my body to tap into its years and years of practice, switch to auto-pilot, and step into the ring.

Three days later, it was time to put my new throwing and breathing techniques to the test. The first round was the qualifying competition. Since it was the home field of my alma mater, I received an extra warm welcome by the packed stadium. I was up against all the big names of the day—Steve Summers, Colin Anderson, Brian Oldfield, and my old friend/nemesis and roommate, Al Feuerbach—plus another ten or so athletes. At least eight of us had a good chance of making the top three, and I was, obviously, a little bit anxious. So what did I do? I breathed.

My first throw surprised me—it felt easy and was legal. Off to a good start. That helped me to relax even more. By the grace of my lucky stars, I managed to qualify the first day—certainly not with a great throw, but one that was good enough.

Next came the finals, with the top eight qualifiers taking six more throws to make the top-three podium and the Olympic team. The other five—and everyone else who had tried without success—would have to wait four more years to try again, or retire. I knew that this was going to be my last attempt at making the Olympics; I'd already been through the wringer plenty, and I'd had enough.

Again, I used those breathing techniques a half hour before the competition, and again it helped. Though the stakes were as high as high could be for this performance, I felt incredibly, unbelievably relaxed. Even my mind was quiet.

Game time. I stepped into the ring, and I simply let the program run. By being calm, I could rely on what I had been pre-programming for my whole athletic life, getting out of my own way and allowing auto-pilot to take over.

I gained the lead by the third throw. Lots of guys were throwing hard, but the shot was going nowhere close to their best distances. Thank goodness. Of course, Al Feuerbach, now the former world record holder (he'd lost his title to a Russian thrower Barishnikov four years earlier) was among the early leaders.

For a while there, we were neck in neck. I took the lead on that third throw, Al took it back on his fourth throw. Then I pulled ahead on my fifth throw. With one more throw left, Al did his best throw of the day—but still he came up a quarter-inch short of mine.

When the final six throws were complete, I leapt up onto the podium, taking first place with the best throw I'd had in the past four years. Coming from my darkest days to being top dog and making my second Olympic team, I stood atop that podium, arm lifted overhead, fist clenched in victory, filled with awe and gratitude. Even though the

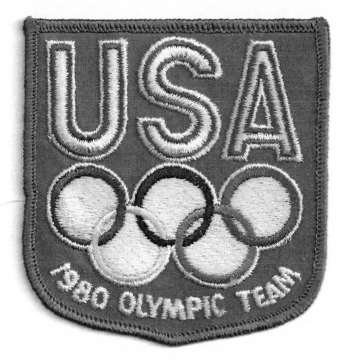

Smile, breathe and go slowly.

THÍCH NHẤT HANH

United States would end up boycotting the 1980 Olympic Games, I felt like I had received a gift more valuable than a chance at gold. It took me a few decades to figure that one out—it wasn't the accomplishment itself, it was all that I'd learned leading up to that moment, and the extraordinary way it had changed my life.

THERE IS POWER IN CALM

Breath is powerful. You know this; you've heard it from Oprah and your doctor and the tomato lady at the farmers' market. Back in 1980, this idea was not as ubiquitous as it is today, and the reason it's taken such a strong hold of our culture since then is not just because it's obvious, but because it's true. There have been tons of studies on breathing and self-regulation, relaxation, digestion, mindfulness, you name it. Now I'm not a pulmonologist or respiratory researcher or free diving champion (those elite athletes can hold their breath for almost twelve minutes!), but I do know from experience that the breath is vital for everything. It's pretty damn simple: no breath, no life. But, in a sense that's more relevant to this story, the breath can help you deal.

Like my football buddies and I discovered (consciously or not) during our pre-game psych-up, the breath changes when we get overly excited, fearful, or anxious. Often it's a chicken-or-egg phenomenon: sometimes the breath induces a difficult emotion, and sometimes an emotion creates a particular breathing pattern. A thought is, of course, part of this formula too. Here's another chicken-or-egg scenario: *What came first, the thought or the emotion?*.

In my athletic career, I found that having an over-stimulated mind interfered with my performance. I'd start with some physical activity that would make me breathe quickly and sporadically, and then my mind would go a little haywire, filling with all those mean, unhelpful, doubting thoughts. My mind would start doing its thing—*Am I ready? Am I strong enough? Am I good enough?*—and that would pull me up into my head and disconnect me from my body. The ripple goes in both directions—in then out, out then in—creating this back and forth conversation between the mind and the body. You can think of it this way: sometimes the mind and the body are speaking different languages, and the breath has to act as the translator. The more in-control the translator, the better the communication. This applies not just to sports, but to any day-to-day situation where you need to be at your best.

When you get up into your head too much, you can use the breath to bring you back down into your body, into your feet. The first thing this does is bring you into the present moment. In his book, *I Am That,* Nisargadatta Maharaj writes, "The past brings regret, the future anticipation." By focusing on your breath, you can center yourself in time, and this allows you to let go of whatever story your mind is chewing on and bring more calm into the body. If you can keep a calm and clear mind, the chance of performing better is greatly increased. You've heard of athletes being "in the zone"—that feeling of time slowing down, of exertion without effort. Breathing meditation slows you down in a way that heightens your ability to pay attention—it'd be much easier to hit the ball if that pitch was coming at you in slow motion, wouldn't it? Then, with this focus and steadiness, your energy—a finite and priceless resource—can be used in a more efficient way to handle anything that life throws at you.

Simple, yes, but not so easy. So how can you get to a more relaxed state? Here's a method that works for me.

PLAY WITH THIS

Find a Quiet Place

Close your office door, silence your phone, tell your kids to go outside. Put aside all distractions. Of course, sometimes it's impossible to eliminate distractions, but no matter. You could do this in the middle of Times Square and still reap the benefits.

Get Comfortable

Sit down or lie down. Loosen your tie, kick off your shoes. Unbutton the top button of your pants (don't worry, nobody's watching). Do whatever you need to do to get comfortable.

Do the Mini Meditation

Take three deep breaths. Focus your attention on the physical sensation throughout, inhaling and exhaling as deeply and slowly as you can. You might pick a physical point to anchor your attention, such as the rise and fall of your chest or belly, the air traveling through your nose, or the movement of air against the skin above your upper lip. Or you could focus on a broader experience of sensation, a whole body type of breathing. Some people even imagine that they are breathing out through the tips of their fingers or toes. It doesn't matter what part you're focused on; play with this and find the right spot for you.

Call Back a Wandering Mind

That's it. It doesn't take very long; depending on how much you've practiced, it'll probably take around thirty seconds. Even so, your mind might wander. If that happens, just bring your attention back to the breath once you realize that that's happening. Don't worry about doing it perfectly—no matter how it goes, whether you were able to stay focused or not, you will benefit. Over time, it'll get easier to keep your mind on the task at hand, to keep it quieter for longer periods. If your mind wanders, no problem; just bring it back. Again, just three breaths.

Do This Practice Again and Again and Again

Try this anytime during your day. I recommend three or four times a day, but if you only do it once, that's a worthy start. A simple way to turn this into a habit is to schedule reminders to go off on your phone throughout the day. Simple. When the alarm goes off, it's time to breathe.

LIFE CHANGING

Not only is meditating on your breath useful for calming the mind before the pursuit of athletic greatness, it's also highly helpful for doing anything in your life better, more efficiently, and with less mental turmoil and greater presence in the moment. This is a good way to prepare yourself when you know that a potentially stressful situation is on its way.

Meditation has been one of the most life changing—if not *the* most life changing—practices I've learned in my life. Like I did before the 1980 Olympic Trials, you can greatly benefit from this breath practice too. It can bring more calm to your day, reduce stress in your life, and give you a greater sense of ease and joy. So make time for the thirty-second breathing before a challenge—no matter what. The more stressful the event, the more you'll need it, and the more you'll be glad you did it.

This is the most important thirty seconds of your day.

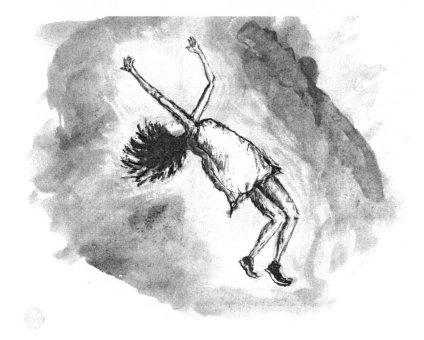

Find ecstasy in life; the mere sense of living is joy enough.

EMILY DICKINSON

INTELLIGENTLY SELFISH

'll be the first to admit it: athletes can be a little self-absorbed. There's really no way around it—if you want to accomplish something specific, time-consuming, difficult, and meaningful, you have to get comfortable dabbling in selfishness. It takes serious focus and considerable discipline to get somewhere, and getting somewhere comes at a price.

So, athletes *have* to be self-absorbed. Most upper-tier athletes get good at making sacrifices and streamlining their processes in order to maximize progress. Over time and with lots of trial and error, athletes will stumble upon/create the best, most efficient routines, systems, sequences, rituals, and methods necessary to achieve their goals. Now, how does that happen? In short: selfishness. Before you begin thinking that I'm suggesting getting all Wall Street–style egomaniacal, we need to add a key word here: *intelligent*. As in, intelligent selfishness. An aspiring athlete has to put him- or herself first, keeping the blinders on to distraction and avoiding the urge to misdirect his or her energy.

For the *life athlete*, the path is not always linear. Goals change, circumstances change, desire shifts. Most folks try something for a while, then discover that, due to new information, it'd be best to try something else. I've been coming back to this point throughout the book: regimen for regimen's sake is not helpful. But regimen for the sake of something bigger, regimen that includes rest and curiosity and flexibility, is an athlete's greatest tool. And to have regimen, you have to set clear boundaries while holding them only until they stop being useful. There are only so many hours in a day, and so we have to be selfish with our time, committing it to something worth investing in.

A friend of mine—a very bright, successful, driven person—had a new goal. His life was quite full and well-organized, and he was one of those guys who naturally made great connections and attracted opportunity. He was set financially, interpersonally, and professionally, but he admitted that something was missing: the ability to do less, to control less in his life. My friend wanted something different. And since he had practice getting things done, he applied his skillset to this new venture. First, he decided that he'd limit his number of activities per day, prioritizing going to the gym, going to work, having dinner with his family, and doing a twenty-minute meditation practice. This opened up the day for him, and allowed him to have more time for rest and relaxation. It's not that he became a hermit or anything like that—instead, every time he was asked to do something beyond these four activities, he'd sit down and really give it some thought before saying yes. He had a purpose and a plan, and the way he went about it was very intelligent, a little bit selfish, and efficient in pointing him in the right direction.

Ultimately, it comes down to freedom; freedom is what you get when you make conscious decisions based on a deliberate plan formulated around what you want to achieve and who you want to be in the world. Sometimes the path is obvious: if you want to ride in the Tour de France, then you better train your ass off, eat right, sleep right, and get onboard with a little (or a lot of) suffering. If you want to get into a long-term relationship, then deal with your issues and stop dating jerks. If you want to learn how to relax, then set the alarm on your phone to remind yourself to breathe. Sometimes the immediate goal is unclear, or it seems a little meandering. But no matter what, if you have some big-picture goal in mind, it's easier to act with intention for the sake of it. To some degree—putting aside forces of nature, the opinions and agendas of others, and your own unrecognized subconscious urges—you rule your world. You have choices to make, so choose wisely.

OUT OF THE RING AND INTO LIFE

The night after the Olympic Trials, I was walking on air. After so much disciplined training, all the athletes were letting loose. The campus was one big party, and after the stressful, high-pressure lead-up to that very unexpected conclusion, I was more than ready to join in. My then-wife was in town to film the movie *Personal Best* with Mariel Hemingway (work which had been launched by her own stint as a hurdler at the 1976 Olympics), and our reunion was tinged with the awkwardness of having spent so much of the last two years apart while I was training.

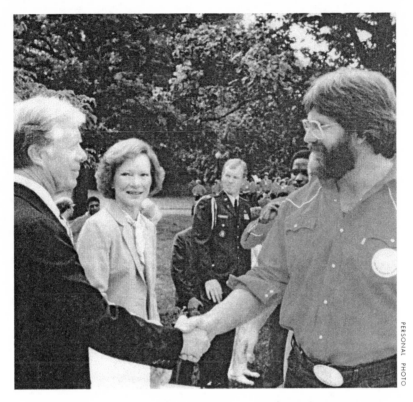

Consolation prize for boycotting the 1980 Olympic Games

Despite our doubts about the future of our relationship, we celebrated together. After she left to go back to work, I kept on partying.

Of course, we athletes had heard warning that the US might boycott the Olympics, and I was aware that a trip to Moscow probably wasn't going to happen. But not going to the Olympics wasn't as big of a deal for me as you might think. Mainly because six weeks prior to the trials, I'd assumed that I had less than a snowball's chance in hell of making the team. My victory was such a big surprise that I really didn't have enough traction for disappointment. Instead, winning the 1980 trials was so deeply satisfying that actually going to the games was barely an afterthought. Of course I would have like to have gone, but quickly it became apparent that it was out of my hands and not worth getting upset about.

I made a stop home in Huntington Beach to get ready to fly with the rest of the new Olympic team for a meet-and-greet with Jimmy Carter at the White House. I think we would all agree that the event was a disaster—all six hundred of us stood in line in that god-awful DC July heat to shake the President's and the First Lady's hands, miserably sweating through our official team attire. It was the start of the 80s, and the outfits were cowboy-themed: I was wearing a thick long-sleeved cowboy shirt, jeans, and boots, plastic soles melting into the grass. I was feeling pretty grumpy about the photo opp as a sorry consolation prize (though I do keep a picture of this moment above my desk—I'm the big guy with the big beard).

After that, I spent one more summer doing what I'd spent a lifetime training for. I competed in Stuttgart, London, Stockholm, Nice—and a handful of other cities I can't remember—earning around $500 a meet. I think my take was something like $4000, and let's just say I didn't feel too guilty about breaking the rules forbidding amateur athletes from getting paid. I'd spent eight years barely scraping by to fund a quashed moment, after all.

My last meet was in Dublin. The shot put had started to feel much heavier than its 16 lb., and so I was a little relieved to say good-bye to my oldest, dearest friend. We'd spent most of my short life together; it was time to move on.

My wife picked me up from the Los Angeles airport. For a day or two I had some hope about patching things up, but it wasn't to be: a few months later she filed for divorce. In the blink of an eye, my marriage and my shot put career were over. And I certainly did not have a plan. I started running on the beach again, surfing, eating less and not even thinking about lifting a weight. I was ready to stop being a big guy, hopeful about learning to move in more dynamic ways.

To pay my bills, I began selling gym equipment in Anaheim while pondering what I was going to do—and who I was in this new era post-jock. I remember at one point right after the trials, I decided to give myself a little time to fall into my new life. *Why not relax for a couple of years, let things take their course?* I thought. Of course, a couple of years turned into a couple of decades.

After a year or so of living in Huntington Beach, I met a beautiful woman from Seattle. My young heart and I believed that she was "the one," so I packed up my Toyota station wagon and, with my sweet pit bull by my side, headed up the I-5 to Washington. During the six months it took for that relationship to peak and die, I got a new job as a trainer—I think that's what my title was, but since this was 1982 and that position wasn't the widely acknowledged and accredited one it is today, I can't be sure. In fact, I was one of the very first people the Seattle Athletic Club hired for this role. My primary duty was to train what felt like a million members on the newest rage: Nautilus equipment. I didn't love my new job, mostly because I knew that there were tons of more functional and efficient exercises out there that could better serve my clients, so to appease my sense of duty to them, I slowly snuck different movements into the "mandatory" Nautilus routine.

One day, a SAC member approached me and said that he recognized me from U of Oregon, where he had been a graduate student and track fan. He just so happened to be a trainer for the Mariners, and he thought I might know how to make a weight-training program that would benefit one of his aging catchers. Rick Sweet was my first non-track pro-athlete client, and we did good work together. Soon Mariners head trainer Rick Griffin noticed our success and hired me to work with the team as their strength and conditioning coach. It was a part-time gig, which I worked for the next eleven years or so. They paid me $50 a game.

Though I was good at what I did, I still worried that training wasn't a "real" profession. Even while working with professional athletes, I kept looking around, trying to find a more acceptable way— from real estate appraisal (which I did for a bit, but wearing a suit and tie plus sitting all day didn't work for me) to fat rendering (an idea which I quickly abandoned)—to earn a living. That started to change as my Mariners work began to attract other top athletes. I worked with pro football and basketball players, PGA golfers, speed boat racers, an Olympic skier, and more. I was able to get them more physically fit and prepared to do their sport, in a way that didn't injure them and—better yet—in which they made constant progress.

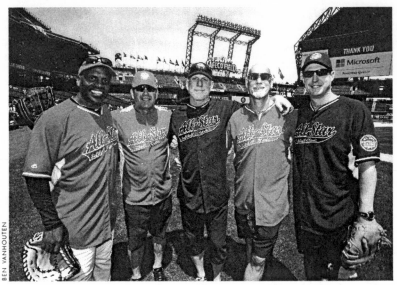

Alvin Davis, Edgar Martinez, Peter Shmock, Jay Buhner, Dan Wilson

Still, despite getting great results, I continued to shrug off any feelings of accomplishment. Back then, trainers—especially those with bodybuilding backgrounds—weren't held in much esteem by more specialized coaches. There was a certain stigma and a particular skepticism, and many of the Mariners players were in this old-school frame of mind. In short, they wanted to play the game, and they thought that in order to improve at playing the game, they simply had to play the game. They feared that weight training would bulk them up and make them "muscle bound," and they didn't do much work outside of the typical hitting and throwing practice. They didn't run or stretch much, either.

Initially, I was often frustrated by my work with the team. I knew that if they trained in the wise, progressive vein of my top-performing track-and-field peers, they would get results, but there remained old myths and strong resistance. There was one player—let's just call him K—who was a gifted athlete and stellar baseballer but not the most open-minded. Every now and then he'd come into the weight room during a session, pick up a weight, make a smartass comment,

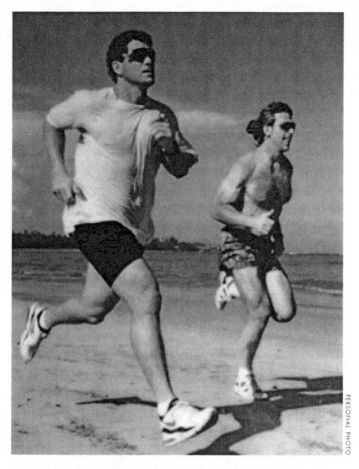

PERSONAL PHOTO

Running with Edgar Martinez on the beach, Puerto Rico, 1993

and leave while looking down his nose at the rest of us. Fortunately, the younger players proved to be more receptive to my ideas. Players like Mark Langston, Edgar Martinez, Alvin Davis, and Jay Buhner were open to giving it a try, and I learned to be content to work with the willing. Randy Johnson, a pitcher now memorialized in the Hall of Fame, really got into the training, even showing up for a yoga practice that I'd arranged with one of my teachers, Mary Forlenza. As time passed and the success of the program spoke for itself, other players began to get on board—and so did their coaches.

But despite this success, a few years into my work with the Mariners, I started to feel lost again. Or rather, the lost-ness I'd been feeling for the past ten years—ever since the end of my athletic career—had finally caught up with me. The training itself was going well, but in my personal life I was making choices that I didn't understand, and that were hurting me and those around me. I'd been through another failed relationship, another failed marriage, and I had a bunch of deep issues and childhood trauma that I really hadn't dealt with. I was a mess—no confidence, and lots of pent-up anger and emotional volatility. The lessons of my athletic career just hadn't fully transferred into my regular life. Basically, after a lot of shit went wrong, I came to a point where I thought: *I don't know why I do what I do.*

JUST IN TIME—THE TEACHER ARRIVES

I heard about Ken Russell from a friend. Born into a Jewish family in Brooklyn, he was seven years my senior, highly opinionated, smart, and sensitive, and he would, in time, come to advocate for me in a way that no one ever had before. He was the teacher I was looking for, the one who was able to lovingly call me on my shit. He was a master of tough love.

For the first couple of years of working with him, I participated in a ten-person group that met once a week at Ken's tidy little house in Woodinville. Then, Ken went off to India to explore himself and the world, and nobody knew if we'd ever hear from him again. When he eventually returned, I started one-on-one work, driving across Lake Washington every week for an individual two-hour session. It was time-consuming and expensive but it was worth it.

Ken was compassionate—and ruthless. He was especially ruthless when looking for the truth. He was the one who formally taught me how to meditate, but that was just a small part of his system of teaching. He directed me to become aware of the ways I habitually deceived myself, and to see how unaware I was when making choices. He helped me discern what was good for me and what situations and relationships were actually making my life less enjoyable and less fulfilling.

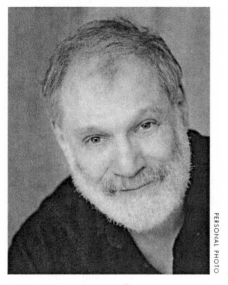

PERSONAL PHOTO

Ken Russell

From him, I learned how to take time off and do self-directed retreats, to live in a more authentic way (which was very uncomfortable at the beginning), and to be quiet. Ken believed that quiet was the key to allowing positive things to come into your life, and through quiet, life could be experienced in a different, fuller way. With more quiet, I had to stop avoiding my shit and stop jumping from experience to experience as a way to distract from negative emotions and difficult memories. I had to learn to be OK with my own company, to be comfortable with myself. It wasn't about pulling away from life—in fact, it was just the opposite. It was about being fully, fearlessly engaged.

Of all the things Ken taught me, the idea of *intelligent selfishness* hit me the hardest. I think he was first to come up with the idea, and now it's a fairly common way to talk about self-care. But it doesn't just apply to single mom social workers who sacrifice everything for everyone else until they become so burnt out and exhausted that their health fails and their lives fall apart. It applies to all of us who want to be more conscious decision-makers, who have committed to a goal or path that requires focus and discipline, who have regular lives and are doing our best to manage them well. Intelligent selfishness is not self-absorption or narcissism or greed—it's simply a way to take care of ourselves so that we can be healthy, happy, and make life work for us. There's that old cliché: if your plane's going down, you have to put on your own oxygen mask before you can help anyone else with theirs.

This teaching was profound for me. Like I've mentioned before, I had spent a lot of time listening to others about how to work out (and how to ignore my body in order to attain a goal). During that first decade post-athletics, I was trying to survive in an unfamiliar world while teaching others at the same time. This lesson of intelligent selfishness was key for me, and one that I would pass on.

Right around this time, and just as my work with the Mariners was wrapping up, I began working with Pacific Northwest Ballet. I was warned that these elite dancers had huge egos, but that was not so—comparing the size of the egos of PNB dancers to the egos of some other professional athletes would be like comparing a single sun to the entire universe. In fact, I encountered little resistance. They were a bit wary at first—there I was, a tall, muscly guy whose best friend had been a big iron ball. "But," I asked them, "throwing a shot put is not much different from a dance, is it?" I then showed them the motion I would do to prepare for a throw. "Same grace, same focus, and same need for calm."

It was a voluntary program, and I trained them like the phenomenal athletes that they were. The way I did my job had changed—I felt more comfortable to articulate all that I'd learned with Ken and others, and so I explicitly concentrated on the mental components of training alongside the physical. Hired to be their "physical and mental performance coach," I focused on creating balance in all realms; it was no different than how I trained other athletes except that we had to be extra careful around making sure they maintained mobility and that the women didn't get bulky, with the addition of having real conversations about the mental and emotional aspects of a career in ballet. Both the men and the women were great at floating gracefully (and making it look easy), so I promoted balance by pushing them to be less "airy." Usually, our workouts would involve plyometric-type exercises and a focus on the center, getting into the feet through the midsection. Then, we'd do a breath meditation. Often we'd end up talking through some drama that had happened during the week, and I would instruct on the strength of a calm mind, how to keep their cool during big performances, and ways to let go of performance mistakes and negative feedback. All that I was learning from Ken about quiet and committing to a way of being I was applying to my work with athletes, and every day underscored each lesson both personally and professionally.

The seeds of the Life Athlete had been planted long before, but now they were really starting to sprout. Based on Bill Bowerman's saying "if you have a body, you're an athlete," it began as a way to encourage folks to think like an elite athlete, to train in a way that would get better, faster results with less effort, sustainable for the long haul. And it extended to the mind—entailing everything I've put here in this book. The Life Athlete philosophy, indebted to a long lineage of smart, disciplined people who have studied and practiced optimal ways to be in the world, was really coming together.

Intelligent selfishness was the final, missing piece. I'd spent a lot of time listening to everyone else about what they thought I should do, and not trusting my own expertise. I'd listened to those mean voices. And I made decisions based on others' needs (or what I thought they needed)—and getting myself in a heap of trouble doing it. This idea was one more method of getting out of the way and approaching life from an internal sense of what was right. It wasn't easy to drop my conditioning—most of us are taught to be nice and polite and say *OK* when we mean *not really*. But, as Ken would say, "This is about making your life work for you, not for everyone else."

I brought this new realization to my athletes; it applies to everyone, including you. It's not about being selfish, it's about making choices grounded in honesty and kindness. You can't help anyone until you put on your own oxygen mask.

PUT YOURSELF FIRST—INTELLIGENTLY

You are the caretaker of your own life. In order to create balance—both internally and out in the world—you need to commit to that role and all the hard work that it entails. Of course, if you're perfectly

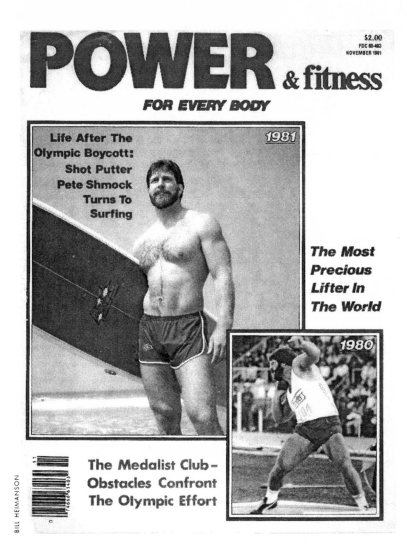

satisfied with your life, then there's no reason to change anything. If, however, there's an area in your life that you want to improve, you have to really focus, weaning yourself from distraction and shedding unnecessary complications. That desire in and of itself reflects intelligent selfishness, as does the actions that spring from it, the drive to develop better habits and a more productive style of thinking. And, for you community-minded folk, don't worry: I'm not suggesting you walk on anyone as you take your own steps forward. Rather, it ripples out. If you feel fresh and vibrant, then you'll do a better job of being a good person and managing your commitments. A healthier you will simply be better at dealing—with work, with family, and with all your other important interests and obligations.

Deciding to be more conscious in the way you organize and take care of yourself ain't easy. Often, it starts with saying no. I must warn you that saying no to that which you've said yes to in the past can be really challenging and uncomfortable. Turning down that perfect cheese Danish for the first time is rough, as is declining an invitation to a late night meetup with friends. If you've been saying mostly *yes* for a while, then your *no* muscle has probably atrophied. But when you set your sights on a goal, you learn how to access your own expertise and follow its direction. It's like doing a pull-up: the first attempt might feel a little pathetic, but you have to start somewhere.

Here are a few everyday examples of intelligent selfishness:

1.   You feel a sore throat coming on. You have dinner plans, and you don't want to be rude by cancelling them (and since you're the center of the universe, you know that your friends will be terribly disappointed). Plus, you hate having that awkward conversation, usually doing anything you can to avoid it. So what do you do? You cancel your dinner plans, go home, heat up some chicken soup, and hit the hay.

2.   You're on a run with a friend, and suddenly you feel a cramp in your calf muscle. But you have this weird competitive thing going with this particular running buddy, and you don't want to feel

like a weenie by admitting to the problem. So what do you do? Question your assumptions about what it means to be a weenie. Are you actually a weenie, or are you just listening to some programing about weenie-ness? You're probably not a weenie. So pay attention to what's really happening—you're just having a cramp—and take care of it. Your friend will understand. In fact, maybe s/he'll take a cue from you and pay better attention next time his or her body is trying to send a message.

3. You have out-of-town guests visiting for a week. Your normal routine sans guests is to go for an hour-long walk every day and to go to the gym twice a week, but you know you'll probably have to change things up while they're around. After four days you've shown them all the tourist hangouts, cooked elaborate meals, eaten more high-end donuts than you've had in the last decade—and not gone on your walks or made it to the gym. Now, you're starting to feel your vitality slide, but you want to be a good host. So what do you do? Tell them that you'd like to go for a walk—you could even invite them to join you. You are not rude for asserting this need, and you don't have to feel guilty for taking a little time for yourself. And if you take this time, you'll feel better and you're guests will get the best of you: fully focused and present, with not an ounce of resentment. Everyone will benefit.

Intelligent selfishness comes from following your body's orders. Remember the "checking in" questions from chapter 3? Ask yourself those. Ask yourself: what can I do right now to be more authentic and live my life in the best way for me?

THE FIVE ELEMENTS NECESSARY TO BE INTELLIGENTLY SELFISH:

Right food
Right sleep
Right movement
Right rest
Right mind/calm mind

Getting these five elements into your life is a daily practice, a practice that focuses you without being regimented. I don't have some magical formula to find your version of "right." No one does. If they say they do, it's up to you to decide if they have an idea based on solid insight, or if they're full of it. Only you know what's best for you, and your body will point you in the right direction. Each one of these elements is part of your practice of being intelligently selfish.

If I boiled down the lessons I've learned throughout my life, it all really comes down to self-care. It's taking the time to ask ourselves big questions and face hard answers, to move toward health and harmony in everything we do. It's about living an engaged, enjoyable, authentic life.

Make your life work for you. This is The Way of the Life Athlete.

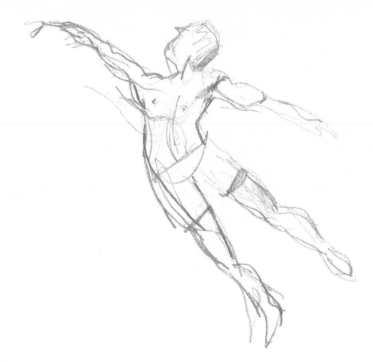

I have to be brutally honest with myself.

JAMIE MOYER, PLAYER, SEATTLE MARINERS

EPILOGUE

I encourage you to remember the following things as you live as a Life Athlete:

> *Without a spark, there can be no fire. I encourage you to want more, to be hungry, to have passion. No matter where you are in your life, there is always room to grow and change. Desire is the catalyst for making that happen.*
>
> *You are powerful. You can't control everything, but there are a lot of things you can practice that will help you to be stronger mentally and physically.*
>
> *Recognize and accept where you are, and move from that place.*
>
> *Follow the cycles of your environment and your body.*
>
> *Work hard, and rest. Be as committed to recovering as you are to working.*
>
> *Seek clarity and calmness.*
>
> *Take care of yourself—you're the only person who can.*

You are a Life Athlete because you are alive and have a body. I encourage you to start living and moving more gracefully and with more strength and vitality right now. I'll be here to cheer you on along the way.

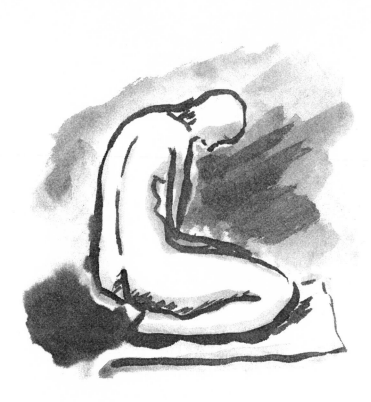

The mind can make a heaven out of hell

or a hell out of heaven

JOHN MILTON

ACKNOWLEDGMENTS

There have been many people in my life who have added to its quality, depth, and meaning. Without their support, encouragement, mentorship, coaching, and good example, I would not have been gifted such wonderful, profound, and life-changing experiences.

The coaches and mentors: Ralph Kroger, Bill Bowerman, The Swim Coach, Tom Tellez, and Ken Russell.

The teachers by way of inspiration and example: Mac Wilkins, Al Feuerbach, Brian Oldfield, Neal Steinhauer, John Powell, the entire track and field crew training in San Jose during 1974–1976, and my dog, Buck.

Those whose support, advice, and dedication keep me going: J Allard, Garth Stein, Peter Bailey, Karen Bryant, Blake Nordstrom, Dan Wilson, Jamie Moyer, and Jeff Ament.

And special thanks to Hank Vigil for his undying support and promotion of *The Way of the Life Athlete* vision.

AUTHOR BIO

Peter Shmock is a two-time Olympian and All-American NCAA track and field athlete. He has worked as a trainer for the Seattle Mariners, the Seattle Reign, the Pacific Northwest Ballet, and many NBA, NFL, and MLB players and Olympic athletes. Mostly he works with average folks who desire to become more vital and physically competent. Peter is the creator of the Elite Edge training class, and now the Life Athlete brand. More info at petershmock.com.

CPSIA information can be obtained
at www.ICGtesting.com
Printed in the USA
FSOW01n2002270816
24183FS

9 780997 656503